Practice Management

Guest Editor

R. REYNOLDS COWLES, Jr, DVM

VETERINARY CLINICS OF NORTH AMERICA: EQUINE PRACTICE

www.vetequine.theclinics.com

Consulting Editor
A. SIMON TURNER, BVSc, MS

December 2009 • Volume 25 • Number 3

SAUNDERS an imprint of ELSEVIER, Inc.

W.B. SAUNDERS COMPANY
A Division of Elsevier Inc.

1600 John F. Kennedy Boulevard • Suite 1800 • Philadelphia, Pennsylvania 19103

http://www.vetequine.theclinics.com

VETERINARY CLINICS OF NORTH AMERICA: EQUINE PRACTICE Volume 25, Number 3
December 2009 ISSN 0749-0739, ISBN-13: 978-1-4377-1281-0, ISBN-10: 1-4377-1281-9

Editor: John Vassallo; j.vassallo@elsevier.com
Developmental Editor: Theresa Collier

Veterinary Clinics of North America: Equine Practice (ISSN 0749-0739) is published in April, August, and December by Elsevier Inc., 360 Park Avenue South, New York, NY 10010-1710. Business and Editorial Offices: 1600 John F. Kennedy Blvd., Suite 1800, Philadelphia, PA 19103-2899. Subscription prices are $222.00 per year (domestic individuals), $339.00 per year (domestic institutions), $111.00 per year (domestic students/residents), $259.00 per year (Canadian individuals), $424.00 per year (Canadian institutions), $224.00 per year (international individuals), $424.00 per year (international institutions), and $151.00 per year (international and Canadian students/residents). To receive student/resident rate, orders must be accompanied by name of affiliated institution, date of term, and the signature of program/residency coordinator on institution letterhead. Orders will be billed at individual rate until proof of status is received. Foreign air speed delivery is included in all *Clinics* subscription prices. All prices are subject to change without notice. **POSTMASTER:** Send address changes to *Veterinary Clinics of North America: Equine Practice*, 3251 Riverport Lane, Maryland Heights, MO 63043. Customer Service (orders, claims, online, change of address): Elsevier Health Sciences Division, Subscription Customer Service, 3251 Riverport Lane, Maryland Heights, MO 63043. Tel: 1-800-654-2452 (U.S. and Canada); 314-447-8871 (outside U.S. and Canada). Fax: 314-447-8029. E-mail: journalscustomer service-usa@elsevier.com (for print support); E-mail: journalsonlinesupport-usa@elsevier (for online support).

Reprints. For copies of 100 or more of articles in this publication, please contact the Commercial Reprints Department, Elsevier Inc., 360 Park Avenue South, New York, NY 10010-1710. Tel.: 212-633-3812; Fax: 212-462-1935; E-mail: reprints@elsevier.com.

Veterinary Clinics of North America: Equine Practice is covered in *MEDLINE/PubMed (Index Medicus), Excerpta Medica, Current Contents/Agriculture, Biology and Environmental Sciences,* and *ISI.*

Printed and bound by CPI Group (UK) Ltd, Croydon, CRO 4YY

Transferred to Digital Print 2011

Contributors

CONSULTING EDITOR

A. SIMON TURNER, BVSc, MS
Diplomate, American College of Veterinary Surgeons; Professor, Department of Clinical Sciences, College of Veterinary Medicine and Biomedical Sciences, Colorado State University, Fort Collins, Colorado

GUEST EDITOR

R. REYNOLDS COWLES, Jr, DVM
Blue Ridge Equine Clinic, Earlysville, Virginia

AUTHORS

EDWARD L. BLACH, DVM, MS, MBA
Dr. Ed, Inc., Monument, Colorado

PETER C. BOUSUM, VMD
President, The Mid Atlantic Equine Medical Center, Ringoes, New Jersey

ANDREW R. CLARK, DVM, MBA
Chief Executive Officer, Hagyard Equine Medical Institute, Lexington, Kentucky

R. REYNOLDS COWLES, Jr, DVM
Blue Ridge Equine Clinic, Earlysville, Virginia

KATHERINE S. GARRETT, DVM
Department of Diagnostic Imaging, Rood and Riddle Equine Hospital, Lexington, Kentucky

MARSHA L. HEINKE, DVM, EA, CPA, CVPM
President, Marsha L. Heinke, CPA, Inc, Grafton, Ohio

BRAD R. JACKMAN, DVM, MS
Diplomate, American College of Veterinary Surgeons, Pioneer Equine Hospital, Oakdale, California

CHARLOTTE LACROIX, DVM, JD
Chief Executive Officer, Veterinary Business Advisors, Inc, Flemington, New Jersey; Assistant Adjunct Professor, University of Pennsylvania School of Veterinary Medicine, Philadelphia, Pennsylvania

GERARD LACROIX, JD, LLM, DEA Droit Sorbonne
Diplomate, Institute d'Études Politiques de Paris, Paris, France

F. RICHARD LESSER, DVM
The Equine Clinic at OakenCroft, Ravena, New York

ROBERT P. MAGNUS, DVM, MBA
President and Chief Executive Officer, Wisconsin Equine Clinic and Hospital; Founder,
Equine Business Management Strategies; Wisconsin Equine Clinic and Hospital,
Oconomowoc, Wisconsin

OWEN E. McCAFFERTY, CPA, AVPM, FACFEI
Owen E. McCafferty, CPA, Inc, North Olmstead, Ohio

CAROL SABO, DVM
Chief of Staff and Owner, Haymarket Veterinary Service, Haymarket, Virginia

TERRY D. SWANSON, DVM
President, Littleton Equine Medical Center, Littleton, Colorado

DENISE L. TUMBLIN, CPA
Wutchiett Tumblin and Associates, Columbus, Ohio

SUSAN H. WERNER, BA
Practice Manager, Werner Equine, LLC, North Granby, Connecticut; Content/
Development Team Member, Rx Works Inc, Las Vegas, Nevada

Contents

Current Economic Trends in Equine Practice   413

Andrew R. Clark

> Current economic trends in equine practice are trends of weakness. Most
> practices, after a decade of double-digit growth, have migrated to survival
> mode within a few months. Understanding that all regions and disciplines
> are affected differently, using the Porter five forces model, we can identify
> changes that must be made in our business models first to survive and
> then to position ourselves to prosper when the recession ends. If we are
> to avoid long-term damage to our practices, we must use cost control
> and work efficiency in addition to price concessions.

Customer Service in Equine Veterinary Medicine   421

Edward L. Blach

> This article explores customer service in equine veterinary medicine. It be-
> gins with a discussion about the differences between customers and cli-
> ents in veterinary medicine. An overview of the nature of the veterinary-
> client-patient relationship and its effects on the veterinarian's services
> sheds light on how to evaluate your customer service. The author reviews
> a study performed in 2007 that evaluated 24 attributes of customer service
> and their importance to clients of equine veterinarians in their decision to
> select a specific veterinarian or hospital. The article concludes with an
> overview of how to evaluate your customer service in an effort to optimize
> your service to achieve customer loyalty.

Gender Shifts in Equine Veterinary Practice   433

Marsha L. Heinke and Carol Sabo

> This article examines gender shifts in equine veterinary practice. A signif-
> icant gender compensation gap continues across the spectrum of profes-
> sions, including veterinary medicine. Many styles of practice serve the
> disparate and sometimes conflicting goals of financial well-being, patient
> care, and physical family presence.

The Transition from Veterinary School to Equine Practice   445

Katherine S. Garrett

> The transition from veterinary school to equine practice can be challeng-
> ing. This article provides suggestions and advice for new graduates in
> areas that include internships, associate positions, financial consider-
> ations, balancing personal and professional responsibilities, mentorship,
> continuing education, and professionalism.

a practice's medical records influence the quality of patient care and client service and affect liability risk, practice productivity, and overall practice value.

This article discusses equine associate employment agreements from the employer's perspective. It should also be of interest to prospective equine associates. The substantive issues and questions are the same, and neither employers nor employees are likely to get far unless they "walk a mile in the other's moccasins".

There are several options to value a veterinary practice (market approach, asset approach, and income approach) and several methods within these approaches. Examples of an income-based approach include excess earnings, discounted future returns, and single period capitalization of earnings. A qualified valuator will use his or her professional opinion and experience to determine the most appropriate method for one's practice situation. This article outlines the excess earnings method for which where the principal components of value are net assets and goodwill.

This article discusses mergers and acquisitions involving equine veterinary practices. Combining practices can be professionally and economically advantageous but requires a great deal of thought, planning, and implementation. If due diligence is performed and true business teamwork is undertaken, the benefits can be enormous and rewarding.

THE CLINICS ARE NOW AVAILABLE ONLINE!

Access your subscription at:
www.theclinics.com

Preface

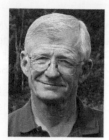

R. Reynolds Cowles Jr, DVM
Guest Editor

This issue discusses practice management and equine practice and comes at a time when our worldwide economy, the horse industry, and equine veterinary practice are suffering through one of the largest financial downturns in recent history. All aspects of the horse industry are in recession, with private sales and consignment sales being off up to 50% in gross and average. Many veterinary practices are reporting a reduction in gross of 10% to 40%. It is imperative that to move through such times, practices must be managed closely in both income production and cost control.

Over the past 10 years, equine veterinary practices have prospered greatly. From the sole practitioner to the large group practices, there has been steady, if not spectacular, growth in all segments of our profession. Many hospitals have been built, and there has been a renewed effort to recruit veterinary students into equine practice. Internships have expanded. Job opportunities have been numerous. All of this has come to a sobering halt in our current economic recession, and none of us can accurately predict when the curve will again turn upward. Equine practice incomes have risen, but expenses, particularly in high-tech diagnostic equipment, have outstripped the income. At times like this, effective management is crucial.

Equine practice has amplified the educational opportunities for veterinarians to increase their knowledge of practice management, and many have taken advantage of these opportunities. The American Association of Equine Practitioners practice management programs, the veterinary management groups, local and state management seminars, more publications on management subjects, and the expansion of qualified equine practice management consultants have all combined to sharpen our management skills.

As you will discover in this issue, the basics of good equine practice are the foundations of economic well-being: practice good medicine and surgery, provide great communications to your clients and staff, conduct your practice in a manner consistent with ethical core values, and combine all of these to deliver great service and value to the horse owner. Using these basics, the equine veterinary community is well positioned to rebound from our current downturn and to prosper in the future. The future will be led by the young practitioner of today who is well educated and trained, is

Vet Clin Equine 25 (2009) ix–x
doi:10.1016/j.cveq.2009.08.001
0749-0739/09/$ – see front matter

compassionate, and delivers individual attention to the horse and its owner. This dedication will result in value for horse owners, and they will reward such attention with economic success for the practitioner.

R. Reynolds Cowles Jr, DVM
Blue Ridge Equine Clinic
4510 Mockernut Lane
Earlysville, VA, USA

E-mail address:
rcowles41@earthlink.net

Current Economic Trends in Equine Practice

Andrew R. Clark, DVM, MBA

KEYWORDS

- Recession • Strategy • Exit Strategy • Meltdown
- Analysis • Return on investment

In May of 2008, when writing an introduction on the topic of "Current Economic Trends in Equine Practice" was assigned to me, it was a fairly straightforward topic on which to write. Economic trends in equine practice have been undergoing a steady and predictable evolution for years. Current Economic Trends in Equine Practice before the late summer of 2008 shaped up like this: all over North America well-managed practices in reasonably strong regional economies had experienced low double-digit growth in gross production for quite a few years. Even equine practitioners who chose, for personal or quality-of-life reasons, to locate their practices in rural regions with depressed economies managed to sustain flat or slight growth despite their geographic choices.

In the months between the late summer of 2008 and the late winter of 2009, the regional, national, and global economies have undergone cataclysmic changes. Historically, the economic trend in equine practice has followed the "rising tide floats all boats" model. Equine practices in general have experienced increased or decreased prosperity in more or less the same ratio. Current trends in equine practice are generally trends of weakness. Unlike our historical trend toward all disciplines rising or falling similarly, the depth of weakness in equine practice is now much more region and discipline dependent. Western discipline practices in Texas and Oklahoma have been more modestly affected by the weak economy, and some continue to prosper. Thoroughbred practices have been decimated by the weak economy. English discipline practices are somewhere in the middle as far as the impact of the weak economy is concerned.

CLIENT EXPECTATIONS

Excellence in technical aspects of equine practice has ceased to be a competitive advantage for a practitioner and has become an expectation on the part of our clients. Technology innovations, coupled with improved training and continuing education

---

Hagyard Equine Medical Institute, 4250 Iron Works Pike, Lexington, KY 40511, USA
E-mail address: aclark@hagyard.com

Vet Clin Equine 25 (2009) 413–420
doi:10.1016/j.cveq.2009.07.006
0749-0739/09/$ – see front matter © 2009 Elsevier Inc. All rights reserved.

opportunities, have contributed to the ability of most equine practitioners to be excellent, thereby fulfilling the expectations of our clients.

PROFIT MARGINS IN EQUINE PRACTICE

The increasing influence and cost of technology, coupled with an industry tendency to undercharge for the use of new technology, has significantly eroded the profitability of equine practices. Before the significant impact of technology on the bottom line, many "average" equine practices generated profit margins in the 30% or greater range. Currently, those margins are in the low teens, and sometimes in the single digits.

EXIT STRATEGY IN EQUINE PRACTICES

Equine practice has suffered under the adage of "you can't sell an equine practice, especially a small one." Without the ability to sell their practice, equine practitioners faced retirement after a dedicated, and often distinguished, career with no exit strategy. This absence of an exit strategy was the product of veterinarians managing their practices like they were jobs instead of businesses. The reality of our profession is that you cannot sell a job that you own, but you can sell a business that you own. In the past decade, there has been a growing migration on the part of equine practitioners from owning jobs to owning businesses. Those businesses have a real value and provide a solid exit strategy for those who choose to manage their practices effectively. A key concept that is critical to understand so as to grasp the current and, more importantly, future trends in equine practice, is the concept of owning a veterinary job versus owning a veterinary business.

To grasp the job versus business concept, one must understand how three terms are used in our analysis; job, business, and good will.

A job is the principal activity in your life that you perform to earn money. A job has no value when you stop working. There is nothing more than the salvage value of instruments and equipment to sell when you stop working at a job that you own.

A business is an organization with the objective of compensating the owner(s) of the practice for the risk they have assumed in addition to compensating people, including the owners, who work as veterinarians in the organization. A business continues to have value when you stop working. You can sell that value (good will) in addition to the salvage value of instruments and equipment.

Good will is an asset of a business. The value of good will is based on the business' established relationships with its customers. Although the asset is intangible, standard accounting practices can be used to calculate a dollar value of the asset.

What's the difference between owning a job and owning a business? A job does not have good will associated with it, whereas a business does have good will associated with it. The value of the good will can be calculated and sold to a successor in the business.

Generations of equine practice owners have owned jobs. The current trend in equine practice is for practice owners to manage toward owning businesses so that they can have an exit strategy.

If you own a job, you have three objectives:

1. Attract and retain customers.
2. Attract and retain staff.
3. Attract and retain associate veterinarians.

If you own a business, you have four objectives:

1. Attract and retain customers.
2. Attract and retain staff.
3. Attract and retain associate veterinarians.
4. Attract and retain new owners for the business.

There are two material factors in the distinction between owning a veterinary job and owning a veterinary business: how much money is made and to whom the money goes.

In terms of how much profit is generated, there are only four fundamental tools for an equine practitioner to use to generate profit: work more hours, cut costs, charge more per hour, and work more efficiently (do more work per hour).

Historically, equine practitioners have relied heavily on the first tool, which is to work more hours. The current trend in equine practice is to begin to understand and use the other three tools: cut costs, charge more per hour, and work more efficiently.

In terms of where the money goes, that is largely a function of your business model and your compensation formula. Job versus business is really determined by the presence or absence of owner compensation (ie, return on investment, excess earnings, profit, bottom line). A business recognizes the difference between compensation earned as an equine practitioner and compensation generated by owning a business. When that line is blurred or nonexistent, the veterinarian probably owns a job instead of a business, and therefore has a weak or nonexistent exit strategy.

A job generates personal earnings sufficient to sustain the practice owner or veterinarian, whereas a business generates personal earnings sufficient to sustain the veterinarian in addition to business entity earnings sufficient to fund a buy or sell transaction. In other words, in a business, the compensation for being the owner of the business should be sufficient to service the debt on the buy-in. More simply, an associate veterinarian who buys in must be paid enough for being an owner to cover the debt service on the buy-in without dipping into his or her veterinary earnings.

IMPACT OF NEW GRADUATES

Current economic trends in equine practice are profoundly affected by the level of interest and preparedness of new graduates.

Interest of New Graduates in Equine Practice

The number of veterinary graduates entering equine practice reached a low point in 2002. An estimate of fewer than 80 of 3500 North American veterinary graduates entered equine practice that year. The myth persisted that "all" equine practices suffered from low pay and poor quality of life.

The reality was that because of inattention to career management and business strategy, some equine practices did suffer from low pay and poor quality of life. Somehow, practitioners in those practices had become the voice of equine practice.

The reality at that time was that many equine practitioners had abdicated the responsibility to speak up about financially successful and high quality-of-life practices. By default, negative and cynical burnt-out practitioners had become the voice of our profession.

A group of equine practitioners engaged in and took charge of their own recruiting in a 2003 event in which 300 third-year veterinary students from North American veterinary schools were invited and had their expenses paid to attend a weekend outing called the Opportunities in Equine Practice Seminar (OEPS). During the weekend, the students heard from 14 energetic and successful North American equine practitioners who told their own stories of financial success and rewarding lives. In addition, the students toured equine hospitals, Thoroughbred farms, and the Keeneland racecourse. The OEPS is now an annual event that garners more sponsorship from equine practitioners, associations, and industry partners and more students each year. In the six years in which the OEPS has been held, there has been an increased focus on the part of the profession on improving compensation and lifestyle issues in those practices that lagged behind in those areas. Also, during that time, the American Association of Equine Practitioners created the Personal and Professional Wellness Task Force to address lifestyle issues. The current status of new graduate interest in equine practice is that in 2008, nearly 200 of 3500 North American veterinary graduates entered equine practice. Increasing the entry of new graduates from 80 to 200 is a huge accomplishment, but is not enough to satisfy the demand for equine veterinary care in the long run.

Preparedness of New Graduates for Equine Practice

For the better part of a century, veterinary medicine has been a four-year curriculum. In the beginning, the time spent on the scientific content of the curriculum, the science of veterinary medicine, was balanced by time spent developing and refining clinical skills, the art of veterinary medicine. The clinical skills time in the curriculum was effective in enabling veterinary students to "get good at" the art of veterinary practice.

As research and science have expanded their place in the veterinary curriculum, the content material related to the art of veterinary medicine, or "getting good at" practice, has been squeezed out of the curriculum. The result is that each generation of graduates knows more and is experienced less than the previous generation of graduates. This has largely transferred the responsibility for clinical experience training (getting good at) to internships in universities and private practice. The shift of caseload away from universities to private referral practices has simultaneously shifted a significant piece of that clinical training responsibility to private practices. It is uncommon for a new graduate veterinarian to enter practice without having completed an internship.

In summary, regarding the preparedness of new graduates entering equine practices, new graduates are better educated and less clinically proficient each year. This is perfectly understandable, given the logarithmic increase in the scientific content packed into the four-year curriculum. The performance gap has been closed by adding internships, often in private practice, as a de facto fifth year of the curriculum.

Gender and Generation Shift in Equine Practice

In Canada and the United States, women constitute approximately 80% of the veterinary college student population.[1] Men are not applying for admission to veterinary colleges to the same extent as women. In the United States, men constituted 44% of the applicant pool in 1985 but only 28% of the applicant pool in 1999.[2] Canada has experienced a similar gender shift in its veterinary student applicant pool.

Each educator, author, and consultant has a theory for explaining the gender shift in veterinary medicine overall and in equine practice specifically. As far as the current state of equine practice is concerned, the reason for the gender shift is less important than the impact of the gender shift. The gender shift is, in reality, a component of the generation shift in equine practice. The high-level impact of the gender and generation shift is the introduction of new practitioners who are unwilling to support the "old school" long-hour and relatively low-pay equine practice model that is associated with practices that function as jobs rather than businesses. The gender and generation shift is responsible for the current trend toward improving the business model of many equine practices. To attract and retain new graduates, equine practices have been pressured to change their business models to improve three components:

1. Work-life balance
2. Compensation
3. Sound ownership transition strategies

The author considers improvement in these three components to be the most important changes to affect equine practice in decades.

INTERNET PHARMACY IMPACT ON CURRENT ECONOMIC TRENDS IN EQUINE PRACTICE

For most of the history of equine practice, equine practitioners have undercharged for professional services and relied on selling pharmaceutics to support their practices. Although a flawed strategy that undermined the value of veterinary service in the marketplace, reliance on pharmaceutic sales kept the equine practice alive for decades.

E-commerce, more specifically, Internet pharmacy evolution, is another source of pressure on equine practice to change the business model. Because the clients of equine practitioners are essentially within a few key strokes of knowing the cost of most products, equine practitioners are forced to discontinue the age-old practice of subsidizing low professional service fees with pharmaceutic sales. There is a tendency for sticker-shock push-back not only from clients, but from seasoned practitioners when faced with the reality of what professional services have to cost to support a viable business model. Practitioners who cling to the low professional service fee model, generally find themselves owning a job rather than a business. This is because clients demand comparable prices to those they see online. Practitioners are left with the choice of losing the client or losing the pharmaceutic sales if they don't react to online pharmaceutic prices. Once the lower pharmaceutic price has been "matched," to sustain profitability, the practice must raise professional service fees to the level they should have been all along. How a practitioner decides to compete with Internet pharmacies is less important than whether or not he or she chooses to continue to undercharge for professional services.

IMPACT OF THE FINANCIAL SYSTEM MELTDOWN

As stated initially, excellence in the technical aspects of equine practice is no longer an advantage; rather, it is an expectation. The current economic trend in equine practice is that to thrive, or perhaps to survive, an equine practitioner must be an excellent equine practitioner and an excellent business manager. The purpose of this issue is to help us become excellent business managers. A good first step in that process is to understand the forces affecting the current economic status in equine practice. There are macro- and microeconomic forces at work in each region and discipline that create significant differences in the relative economic strength or weakness in equine practices.

The macroforces affecting equine practice at the time of this writing (first quarter of 2009) largely relate to four factors:

1. The impact of the equity market on the net worth of clients
2. The effect of extremely tight credit on practices, clients, and suppliers
3. The depressed market value and inability to sell real estate
4. The depressed market value and difficulty of selling horses

The microforces at work in various regions and disciplines are conveniently evaluated with a strategy known as Porter's Five Forces Analysis. While affiliated with the Harvard Business School, Porter outlined a framework for industry analysis and business strategy looking at five forces that determine the attractiveness of an industry:

1. The bargaining power of suppliers
2. The bargaining power of buyers
3. The intensity of rivalry
4. The threat of new entrants
5. The threat of substitutes

Using these five forces, Porter estimates the attractiveness of an industry. Porter defines attractiveness as the overall industry profitability. An "unattractive" industry is one in which the combination of forces acts to drive down overall profitability. An unattractive industry would be one approaching "pure competition" or commodity status.[3]

Because one size does not fit all with regard to the current economic situation in equine practice, it is this author's suggestion that we use Porter's five forces as a checklist to understand the microenvironment affecting the current trends in the specific market in which each of us works. To facilitate the reader's use of the Porter model, the author describes how he believes it applies to equine practice.

Porter's five forces examine forces on a practice that affect its ability to attract and maintain customers and generate profit. A change in any of the five forces requires or enables a practice to change its business strategy. A diversified practice may need to have several "Porter's five forces" analyses to assess its overall situation accurately.

Porter's five forces include three forces from horizontal competition (the threat of substitute products, the threat of established rivals, and the threat of new entrants) and two forces from vertical competition (the bargaining power of suppliers and the bargaining power of customers).[3]

Threat of Substitute Products

In equine practice, there is not a genuine substitute product for veterinary care, but there are a plethora of products and services that horse owners substitute for veterinary care. This "try everything else before you call the vet" approach in an attempt to save money, often yields little else but a diminished horse owner budget. Our most useful tool in combating the threat of substitution is horse owner education.

Threat of the Entry of New Competitors

Attractive markets that yield high returns draw equine practitioners. This eventually decreases profitability. There is no legal or ethical way to block these new practitioners from entering the market to ensure that the profit rate declines towards a commodity level.

Established well-managed equine practices can mitigate the impact of new competitors by managing their "brand." A brand is the identity every practice has and every practitioner has. You may choose to manage your brand, or you may choose not to manage your brand. Either way, you have a brand. Emphasizing personal brand over practice brand, generating client loyalty to a person rather than loyalty to a practice, creates an opportunity for new competitors to "poach" clients. If clients are only loyal to one practitioner in a practice rather than to the practice, they are more likely to switch to a new provider of veterinary care.

Intensity of Competitive Rivalry

In equine practice, the intensity of competitive rivalry is usually the primary contributing force to the unattractiveness (low profitability) of a region or discipline. Although some practices compete on non–price-related levels, such as marketing and service, there is certainly a tendency in equine practice for rivals to compete aggressively on price. We see the "commodity strategy" in the midst of the current economic downturn in central Kentucky. A few practitioners who have elected to use this strategy drive into farms with the offer, "whatever your vet charges, I will charge less…a lot less." This behavior is partially fueled by the relative equine practice overcapacity as demand for equine practice veterinary services shrinks (see section on threat of the entry of new competitors).

Bargaining Power of Customers

The ability of customers to put the practice under pressure and the customer's sensitivity to price changes are two characteristics of a region or discipline in which there is unusual power in the hands of the customers. This force is magnified in a region or discipline in which equine practitioners have chosen to compete on price.

Because the client's expectation is excellence from the equine practitioner, the customer perceives there to be little disadvantage associated with switching to a new veterinarian on the basis of price.

The customer's sensitivity to price change is a measure of the "elasticity of prices." As the price of a good or service increases, consumers usually demand a lower quantity of that good or service. They may consume less of that good or service or substitute it with the same good or service from a lower cost provider. The greater the extent to which demand decreases as price increases, the greater is the price elasticity.[4]

Bargaining Power of Suppliers

Suppliers of drugs, supplies, components, and services (eg, expertise) to the practice can be a source of power over the firm. The bargaining power of suppliers is essentially a supply and demand issue. In the past decade, the largest impact from the bargaining power of suppliers was in the relative lack of veterinarians entering equine practice. In the midst of the current economic downturn, the demand for veterinary services is decreasing; thus, the power of suppliers (new graduates) may, in fact, be diminishing.

SUMMARY

Current economic trends in equine practice are trends of weakness. Most practices, after a decade of double-digit growth, have migrated to survival mode within a few months.

Understanding that all regions and disciplines are affected differently, using the Porter model, we can identify changes that must be made in our business models first to survive and then to position ourselves to prosper when the recession ends.

We must avoid fear-based decision making regarding pricing. Equine practitioners have struggled for the better part of 15 years to get prices to reflect not only the cost of providing veterinary care but to provide a meaningful return on investment to practice owners. That return on investment to practice owners is critical to any succession plan or exit strategy. If equine practitioners choose to slash prices as a primary strategy to survive, our profession is destined to relive the 15-year struggle to get our business models sound. If we are to avoid long-term damage to our practices, we must use cost control and work efficiency in addition to price concessions.

REFERENCES

1. Summary of the proceedings at the 2002 summit meeting considering the report of the CVMA Task Force on: education, licensing, and expending the scope of veterinary practice. Can Vet J 2002;43:755–7.
2. Slater MR, Slater M. Women in veterinary medicine. J Am Vet Med Assoc 2000; 217:472–6.
3. Porter ME. Competitive strategy, techniques for analyzing industries and competitors.
4. Available at: http://en.wikipedia.org/wiki/Elasticity_(economics). Accessed February, 2009.

Customer Service in Equine Veterinary Medicine

Edward L. Blach, DVM, MS, MBA

KEYWORDS

- Customer • Service • Client • Veterinarian
- Veterinarian-client-patient relationship

Veterinary medicine is a profession and a business. It requires dedication and discipline to learn and apply a specialized body of knowledge. In most cases, however, applying that knowledge with interest or attention only to the details of the profession or discipline, and without attention to the details of capturing value from the application of that knowledge, yields a short life span in the profession. If you apply your professional knowledge without taking care of the appropriate business processes with which value is captured, you may have a short-lived career or a poorly performing practice.

Veterinarians are expected to have a minimum level of expertise and competence in applying veterinary medical procedures. Competence is the expected minimum criterion for every veterinarian. It is no longer a competitive advantage. Thus, veterinarians must compete on the basis of criteria by which they can differentiate themselves from the rest of the profession, and one of the most important differentiators is customer service.

Traditionally, most veterinarians have little training in business and customer service because their education focused primarily on the attributes of providing sound veterinary decision making. Perhaps one reason why veterinary medicine has not "spoken" frequently about customer service historically is the conflict between the words "customer" and "client." Many professionals profess that they have clients rather than customers. This dilemma does not have to impair the veterinarian's ability to provide optimal service. Instead, if the veterinarian acknowledges that clients have a choice regarding the selection of their veterinarian similar to that of customers in other industries, the services offered by the veterinarian can be provided with the customer's preferences clearly at the center of the process. Assessing the differences in the definitions and related perceptions about client versus customer should help to develop the right philosophy with which to evaluate and develop optimal customer service criteria for your practice.

Dr. Ed, Inc., PO Box 1341, Monument, CO 80132, USA
E-mail address: ed@dr-ed.com

Vet Clin Equine 25 (2009) 421–432
doi:10.1016/j.cveq.2009.07.001
0749-0739/09/$ – see front matter © 2009 Elsevier Inc. All rights reserved.

vetequine.theclinics.com

The term *client* is defined as "the party for which professional services are rendered".[1] The term *customer* is defined as "a person who purchases goods or services from another".[2] When studying these definitions, it becomes obvious which definition is more useful when evaluating how you serve your clients. The definition for client indicates that something is done for or to the client by the professional, almost with an attitude that "the person is lucky I'm here for him or her." In contrast, the definition for customer indicates that the person purchasing the product or service is the decision maker in the process, the one who must be satisfied. With these definitions in mind, it is helpful to develop a customer-oriented philosophy within your professional service business. By developing a customer-focused service and culture, you may find that members of your team are likely to look for and implement ways to serve your clients more like customers. For purposes of this article, the term *customer* is used when discussing how you serve (ie, customer service) and the term *client* is used when discussing whom you serve, as a show of respect for the people you serve.

WHAT IS CUSTOMER SERVICE?

What is customer service? Customer service represents all the attributes of how you serve your clients. It is the experience that you provide your clients when they choose to do business with you, and they do choose. The technical component of your service is only a small part of what your clients want and expect when they seek your help. In a service business, customer service, or the customer experience, is your brand. It is your identity. It defines who you are to your clients and your marketplace. The word "brand" comes from the Norse word "brandr," which means "to burn".[3] Your brand is the identity or image that is burned into the minds of your clients and the rest of your market. It is the promise that you make to your clients, and it defines the service(s) that you provide.

Customer service in veterinary medicine is complicated by the nature of the relationships that exist in the ordinary transaction. In veterinary medicine, there is a patient and there is a client, and both require different types and levels of service to achieve satisfaction. There is a triangular relationship (**Fig. 1**), and all parties must be served optimally to achieve the desired result of an extremely satisfied customer.

It helpful to visualize the relationships that must be managed by the veterinarian, because the needs of the customer and the patient are different yet closely related. There are separate and distinct attributes of your customer service that are designed for the patient, and others are specifically designed for the client. Therefore, when

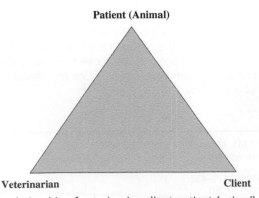

Patient (Animal)

Veterinarian   Client

Fig. 1. The triangular relationship of veterinarian-client-patient (animal).

evaluating your customer service, it is helpful to segment all aspects of the service that you provide with specific detail toward the patient and the client. For example, in **Box 1**, the matrix illustrates what might be important to each party in the interaction with the veterinarian in the typical veterinarian-client-patient encounter.

In reviewing the attributes of each party in the veterinarian-client-patient relationship, it is apparent that there are synergies between and among the participants in this interaction. It is also possible to see that the patient and client have different perspectives in the interaction, both using different senses to assess and manage their positions in the triangle. It is this different perspective and the requirement to use different senses attributable to their differing abilities that make it important to address the patient experience separately from the client experience in the typical veterinarian-client-patient interaction. For example, the veterinarian communicates with the patient by means of posture, tone of voice, manner of handling, and other nonverbal communications. At the same time, the veterinarian communicates with the client by means of verbal communication in addition to the physical and postural communications that are sensed by the patient and the client. Thus, different senses are used by the patient and client in communicating with the veterinarian. The veterinarian must be cognizant of these differences and proactively manage the veterinarian-client-patient relationship in a manner that satisfies each party.

PATIENT EXPERIENCE

The patient experience is the part of the service that veterinarians invest years in school learning to perfect. The patient in veterinary medicine is the animal. Thus, the patient experience involves all the following:

- Patient handling
- Patient care
- Diagnostic procedures and processes
- Treatment procedures and processes
- Medical outcome

The patient experience represents that part of the service that veterinarians are more comfortable in valuing when they establish and implement their fee schedule. This does not mean that the values are appropriately established, but the scientific and procedural technique-based part of veterinary services is clearly the area of focus for most veterinarians when it comes to delivering service and capturing value in return.

It is important to consider the relationship between the patient and client when establishing your service parameters and processes. If the animal is perceived by the client to be a member of the family, the client expects you to treat the patient with a level of care that resembles respect for a family member. If you do anything to denigrate the "value" or importance of the patient in any way, your brand is devalued as well. Conversely, if the patient is one that plays an economic role in the life of the client, it is important that you at least consider the economic implications of your recommendations and communicate those implications clearly to your client.

What typically happens in equine veterinary medicine is that the veterinarian often makes judgments regarding client preferences and desires for patient care based on economic implications when the client may be more concerned with the implications of the challenges the illness has on his or her relationship with the patient rather than with the economic implications. This judgment is probably rooted in the historically agrarian background of many veterinarians. This often results in the client being

Box 1
Attributes of the veterinarian, client, and patient

Attributes of the patient

Needs and receives the diagnostic or treatment

Cannot talk

Feels the pain or discomfort

Uses all senses to assess the situation

Uses nonverbal communication

Important to the patient

I'm ill and need your help.

I have a desire to get well.

Is the environment safe?

Is this going to be painful?

Does the medicine taste good?

Are there other animals nearby?

Is the environment pleasing?

Am I hungry?

Am I frightened?

Am I safe?

Attributes of the client

Has emotional connection to the patient

Is responsible financially for the services being sought

Cannot feel the pain but is sensitive to the fact that the patient does

Can communicate verbally with the veterinarian

Important to the client

My patient is ill. I want it to get well.

Is the environment clean?

Is the environment safe?

Are the people nice?

Do the people respect me?

Do the people respect and care for my patient?

Is the patient getting better?

Is the patient's pain being prevented or managed?

Did the people do all that they could do?

How much will this cost?

Are there going to be any surprises?

Do I understand everything?

Has the communication been thorough?

Is it easy to get what I want?

Attributes of the veterinarian

Cannot communicate verbally with the patient

Can talk to the client

Must manage the patient

Must manage the client

Must manage the business and the medicine without conflict

Important to the veterinarian

Did I make the right diagnosis?

Did I perform the procedure to the best of my ability?

What does the client want?

Is the client happy?

Is the patient getting better?

Am I going to get paid?

What else am I responsible for today?

---

less than fully satisfied because he or she may perceive that the veterinarian does not care or is not sensitive to the fact that the patient is a member of the family rather than an economic priority or commodity.

CLIENT EXPERIENCE

The client experience is the most challenging part of the veterinary-client-patient encounter for several reasons. First of all, selection committees to veterinary schools have historically selected heavily toward students with a passion for animals rather than a passion for serving people. In fact, many veterinarians admit to pursuing veterinary medicine because of their preference for working with animals rather than people. In fact, veterinary medicine is a predominantly people-oriented profession. We must build a team of people who are dedicated to serving the needs of people with animals. Fortunately, compassion for animals and compassion for people are not mutually exclusive qualities. As most surveys attest, the general public holds veterinarians in high esteem, primarily because of the compassion and care that they exhibit for their patients and clients.

In addition, veterinary students have historically received little instruction regarding managing a team of people or the client relationship, because there is little time in the curriculum for nonscientific teaching. This fact makes it even more important for veterinarians to surround themselves with high-quality people selected for their skills and demeanor to serve their clients optimally.

The client experience includes all aspects of your service from the first contact seeking service or information, through the process of obtaining care for the animal, to the follow-up necessary to complete the care. What do your clients experience when they decide to use your veterinary services?

It is recommended that you map your clients' journey through their experience with all areas of your service.[3] Map every point of contact of your customers with your brand or service. How did they learn about you? What do they experience when they seek more information? Is their experience a positive one with your Internet presence? Is their reception on the telephone effective, friendly, and representative of the level of care that you want to provide? What do they experience when they arrive at your clinic? Is the environment clean, safe, and pleasing? Are the directions well defined? Are they welcomed and greeted when they arrive? Do they have to wait long to see the doctor? Does the doctor have all the information and tools to provide optimal service? Does the client feel that the doctor spent adequate time explaining and educating him or her? Did the veterinarian handle the patient with compassion and care? Were treatment instructions clear? Were the costs and timelines of treatment well defined in advance? Was the client satisfied with the follow-up? Do you know the level of satisfaction with the patient care, client service, and medical outcome? What sources of information do your clients use when they have a question? How do they prefer to communicate? Would they recommend your service to their friends? Are they likely to use your service again?

All these questions should be thoroughly evaluated in your process of mapping your customers' journey through your service. By doing this, you and your team put yourselves in the position that your clients face when they use your services.

What do Clients Want?

To develop optimal customer service, it is imperative that veterinarians understand what their clients want from their veterinary service. It is also important to develop an understanding for the preferences of clients when they select a veterinarian to provide animal care. Clients of veterinarians have expectations and preferences regarding how veterinary services are provided; however, before a study conducted in 2007,[4] it was unknown how well equine veterinarians understood the expectations and preferences of their clients. Clients make decisions to select their veterinary service provider based on many criteria, only one of which is the competence of the veterinarian, and even then, customers have little training in judging the competence of veterinarians.

In the summer of 2007, a study was designed and implemented to look at the level of importance of a variety of criteria in a client's decision to hire a specific veterinarian or veterinary clinic.[4] These results were compared with equine veterinarians' perceptions regarding what they believed was most important in clients' decisions to hire a specific veterinarian or clinic. An overview of the study follows.

The questionnaire was designed to determine the level of importance to horse owners of 24 different criteria that are a part of the overall service experience provided by equine veterinarians. These same criteria were presented to equine veterinarians for their ratings of the level of importance that they perceived clients place on each of the criteria.

The veterinary questionnaire was sent to the US membership of the American Association of Equine Practitioners (AAEP) by means of e-mail. The horse owner questionnaire was sent to approximately 15,000 horse owners who had previously enrolled in the AAEP Owner Education Program for their input. The questionnaire was developed and presented using the Zoomerang.com system of market research and analysis.

Horse owner responses

One thousand two hundred seventy-three horse owners responded to the questionnaire. The respondent profile was within expected limits for the industry with respect to breed, discipline, gender, age, and state.

Veterinary responses

Five hundred ninety-eight AAEP-member veterinarians completed the online questionnaire using the Zoomerang.com system. The respondent profile was within the normal expected limits of the equine veterinary population in the United States.

Results

The average responses regarding the level of importance for each customer service criterion for horse owners and veterinarians are shown in **Fig. 2**, with the criteria in descending order of what was most important to horse owners to what was least important to horse owners. Average veterinary responses to the same criteria ratings are shown side by side with the horse owner responses.

Horse owners gave all 24 criteria an average rating of at least 3.5 of 5.0, indicating that all criteria carried some positive level of importance in their overall experience and expectations for service from the equine veterinarian. Eighteen of 24 criteria received average ratings of at least 4.0 of 5.0 by horse owners. Thus, it is important to take all these criteria seriously when reviewing your service offerings.

As expected, horse owners selected "competence in veterinary skills" as their most important criterion when selecting a veterinarian. It was obvious from the general comments of veterinary respondents that there was significant skepticism regarding horse owners' abilities to judge the competence of the veterinarian. Competence is difficult to define, but there are some insights in the data that may help to define what clients really mean.

First of all, as expected, after "competence," horse owners selected criteria that could collectively be classified as relating to interpersonal skills of the veterinarian or the general outcome of their experience with the veterinarian or clinic. In the absence of sound criteria for judging competence, clients use what we all use when

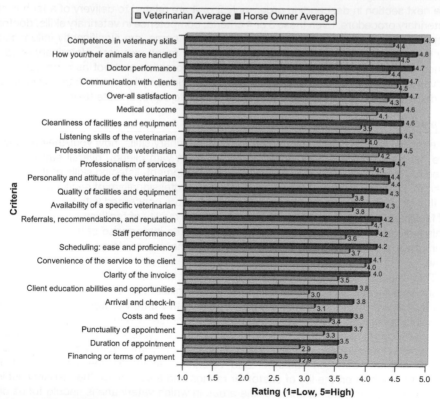

Fig. 2. Customer service ratings: veterinarians versus horse owners.

judging the service we receive. We see how clearly the service provider communicates with us in educating us about what to expect, listening to our concerns, and communicating the findings or expected outcomes of our experience. Even if the outcome is not our preference, if the service provider has done everything he or she can to optimize the outcome or to deal appropriately with the challenges we have presented and he or she has treated us with care and respect, we are most likely satisfied with the service and are likely to go back in the future.

Regarding interpersonal skills of the veterinarian, "how they handled my horses" is the number one interpersonal skill of the veterinarian, in that a veterinarian's manner of dealing with patients is an indicator to clients regarding how much they care for the patient and, in turn, the client. It is important to remember that horse owners would not bring their horse to the veterinarian if there was not a significant amount of "care" and emotional investment already in place.

"Communication with clients" and "listening skills of the veterinarian" provide an additional indication of the importance that clients place on interaction with their veterinarian. This interaction must take the form of complete communication, which includes strong listening skills. Listening communicates to the client the level of care and respect that the veterinarian has for him or her.

Furthermore, highly rated criteria, such as "doctor performance," "overall satisfaction," and "medical outcome," are all closely related to the overall experience of how the client and the patient were treated in their experience with the veterinarian and his or her staff.

When looking at the top 10 most highly rated criteria by horse owners, as shown in the next section in descending order, only 3 or 4 are related to delivery of a technical veterinary procedure. Even these 3 or 4 criteria, competence in veterinary skills, doctor performance, overall satisfaction, and medical outcome, are significantly influenced by the interpersonal skills of communicating how much you care. Veterinary excellence must be assumed as a minimum to be in practice and not as a competitive advantage. Competitive advantage is now determined by how veterinary excellence is delivered and how much veterinarians are able to communicate their level of care.

Top 10 Service Criteria

The top 10 service criteria are competence in veterinary skills, how your/their animals are handled, doctor performance, communication with clients, overall satisfaction, medical outcome, cleanliness of facilities and equipment, listening skills of the veterinarian, professionalism of the veterinarian, and professionalism of services.

It is also worth noting that horse owners were more concerned with the cleanliness of facilities and equipment than they were with the quality of facilities and equipment. This indicates that we should not underestimate the importance of how we present ourselves, our facilities, and our equipment whether we are large or small or old or new.

This discussion would not be complete without emphasizing that nowhere to this point have we discussed "costs and fees" as a significant determinant of how a horse owner selects a veterinarian or a clinic, because this criterion was rated 21st of 24 possible service criteria in level of importance by horse owners.

It is important to consider not only which criteria customers viewed as more important versus the criteria that veterinarians viewed as most important but the magnitude of the disparity between customer and veterinary ratings for the same criteria. If criteria were high on the list of customer ratings and also high on the disparity list in **Fig. 3**, it is an indicator of some of the areas in which veterinarians should focus on improving customer service.

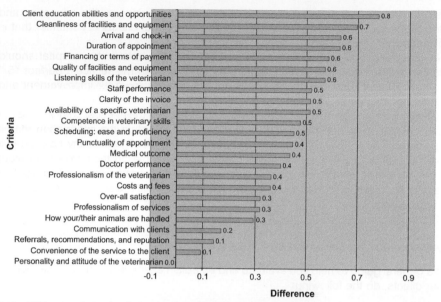

Fig. 3. Difference between horse owner and veterinarian ratings.

Veterinarians, on average, rated all criteria lower in importance than did horse owners, with the exception of "personality and attitude of the veterinarian." This may be an indication that horse owners place a higher level of importance on customer service, in general, compared with the veterinarians who serve them.

In summary, the following recommendations can be made when reviewing your customer service offering:

1. Assume veterinary excellence is a minimum rather than a competitive advantage.
2. Customers want to know how much you care.
3. Communicate how much you care in all that you do for your clients—not just in words but in how you present yourself and your services. Listening communicates care. Even the cleanliness of your facilities, equipment, and people conveys clearly how much you care, and clients notice.
4. Educate your entire team about how everything they do communicates to the client how much you care and that this is your brand.

ACHIEVING OPTIMAL CUSTOMER SERVICE

What should be the goal regarding customer service? Is the goal to have satisfied customers or loyal customers? Fred Lee,[5] in his book entitled *If Disney Ran Your Hospital*, suggests that loyal customers should be the goal. He suggests that satisfied customers do not necessarily use only your services or recommend you unconditionally to their friends and colleagues. He suggests that only the most loyal and most satisfied customers recommend you unconditionally. He recommends that your service should be "memorable" to the client. It should create an experience that surpasses the client's expectations of normal. Your service should provoke story-telling from a client when your service comes to mind. These exemplary memories are created by having a team and company culture that goes above and beyond what is expected. Do you go out of your way to comfort your stressed clients when their horses are experiencing illness or discomfort? Do you provide education and information beyond what they expect? Do you thank your clients in a manner that is not ordinary?

In assessing customer service ratings, Lee[5] recommends that a hospital should assume that the only loyal customers are those who rated the service a perfect "5." Any rating lower than a perfect 5 suggests that there is room for improvement and that if customers find a service that is a perfect 5, they are likely to try it.

Clients want you, as their service provider, to anticipate their needs. They should not have to navigate a maze of people and processes to obtain the information that is important to them. How easy is it to do business with you? How many calls does it take for clients to get what they want? How many people do they have to contact to get what they want? How long does it take them to receive service or results? All these questions should help you to determine how well you are anticipating the needs of your clients.

SUMMARY: HOW TO BUILD YOUR CUSTOMER SERVICE TEAM

As a general guide to help you evaluate and establish exemplary customer service for your clients, do the following:

1. Have all your key team members read the book entitled *Good to Great* by Jim Collins.[6] This group exercise can help you to develop a company culture that is focused on teamwork and accomplishing extraordinary results.
2. Make this recommendation from Dr Andy Clark, DVM, MBA (personal communication, 2005) the foundation for your service to your clients:
    a. Never surprise them.
    b. Never frustrate them.
    c. Never make them call you back.
        Note: If your team follows these three simple promises to your clients, they may find many ways in which you are not currently serving your clients optimally. They can also use these principles as a guide for immediate intervention when necessary, and when they do, your clients should be greatly amazed. Their experience should be memorable.
3. Map the client's journey with your team.
    a. Map the client's journey when using your services.
        i. Would you be satisfied if this was your journey as a client?
        ii. Is the client's journey compatible with his or her expectations according to his or her relationship with the patient?
    b. Map the patient's journey when using your services.
        i. Ensure that the patient's journey is compatible with a positive experience for the client as well.
        ii. Does the patient's journey communicate respect and care for the client and the patient?
4. Define your brand promise.
    a. Evaluate every facet of what you communicate to your clients about your services.
        i. How you present yourself and your practice
            (1) Attire, vehicle, facilities, equipment, cleanliness
            (2) Business cards, stationary, branding, invoices
            (3) How the telephone is answered, responsiveness
            (4) Fees, operational processes, your team

(5) How easy is it to do business with you?
    a. For what are you known?
    b. What is your promise to your clients?
    c. How do you keep your promise?
    d. How much do you care?
    e. How do clients know how much you care?
    f. Have you watched how your clients use your services?
    g. What is their experience?
    h. Have you asked them?

5. Build your team.
    a. Recruit people for the role they are going to play in your company. Hire friendly, compassionate, and smart people.
    b. Recruit people with the specific skill set that you need or the capacity and motivation to learn it.
    c. Train your team.
    d. Empower your team. Let them serve. Do not require them to get your permission to serve your clients optimally and immediately.

6. Provide incentives for complete team performance.
    a. What you measure is what drives your team.
      i. Ensure that the incentives are designed to motivate a specific behavioral result. Incentives work; thus, be certain that what you are motivating is exactly what you want.
      ii. If you only measure efficiencies, your team is likely to place more importance on achieving efficiencies at the expense of serving your clients.
      iii. Discuss episodes of customer service failures with your team. Ask them to remember any time when they were the customer and the service was so poor that they came away from the experience totally exasperated and angry. Have them share those episodes with their fellow team members. After all team members have the opportunity to share these episodes, ask them what all these examples have in common. Unconditionally, all these episodes have in common the fact that the service provider did not care. By completing this exercise, you can successfully put your team members in the shoes of your clients. They should begin to realize and share examples of how they can go beyond normal to create memorable experiences for your clients.

By following these general guidelines, you should be able to build a team that is highly focused on delivering a memorable client-focused service to your clients and patients. This is the foundation for developing a growing veterinary enterprise that delivers veterinary services in an optimal manner to a group of increasingly loyal clients. The result should be a more profitable and valuable enterprise and a more enjoyable, satisfying professional experience.

REFERENCES

1. Client. (n.d.). Dictionary.com unabridged (v. 1.1). From Dictionary.com Web site. Available at: http://dictionary.reference.com/browse/client. Based on the Random House Dictionary, Random House, Inc, 2009. Retrieved March 21, 2009.
2. Customer. (n.d.). Dictionary.com unabridged (v. 1.1). From Dictionary.com Web site. Available at: http://dictionary.reference.com/browse/customer. Based on the random house dictionary, Random House, Inc, 2009. Retrieved March 21, 2009.

3. Adamson AP. BrandSimple. New York: Palgrave MacMillan; 2006. p. 30, p. 137–46.
4. Blach EL. Client communications: the importance of customer service in equine practice. American Association of Equine Practitioners Proceedings of the 2007 Practice Management Seminar. Lexington (KY), July 27–30, 2007.
5. Lee F. If Disney ran your hospital. Bozeman (MT): Second River Healthcare Press; 2004.
6. Collins J. Good to great. New York: Harper Collins Publishers; 2001.

Gender Shifts in Equine Veterinary Practice

Marsha L. Heinke, DVM, EA, CPA, CVPM[a], Carol Sabo, DVM[b],*

KEYWORDS

- Gender • Compensation • Labor • Economics • Women
- Practitioner • Veterinarian • Trends

WOMEN AND WORK IN THE UNITED STATES

The iconic World War II image of "Rosie the Riveter" presages the economic force of women in all facets of the American workplace, including the veterinary profession. From 1940 to 1944, the number of working women jumped 57%,[1] and they filled every aspect of work opportunities, not just factory positions. The patriotic call of duty to all citizens, and women's answer to it, forever changed our understanding of the ability of women to perform well in the work force.

After World War II, women remained in the work force but shifted primarily to clerical and administrative positions. The next great influx of women into the work force did not occur until the 1970s.

The first female veterinarian graduated from Cornell University in 1910.[2] The first survey of the American Association of Veterinary Medical Colleges in 1968 to 1969 showed that women comprised 8% of the total US veterinary college student body.[3] Not until the mid-1970s did the number of women accepted to veterinary colleges increase substantially.

The watershed year of 1986 to 1987 saw women achieve a 53% proportion of all veterinary college students. The number of female veterinarians in practice has steadily increased, reaching 50% of the American Veterinary Medical Association (AVMA) membership in 2007.[4] The current proportion of female equine practitioner members of the American Association of Equine Practitioners (AAEP) is 42.4% (N. Altwies, Membership Services Coordinator of the American Association of Equine Practitioners, personal communication, 2009).

Many factors have contributed to the gender shift experience in general and in the veterinary profession specifically. Some commonly cited reasons include the following:

---

[a] Marsha L. Heinke, CPA, Inc, 934 Main Street, Grafton, OH 44044, USA
[b] Haymarket Veterinary Service, PO Box 1005, Haymarket, VA 20168, USA
* Corresponding author.
E-mail address: haymarketvet@aol.com (C. Sabo).

Vet Clin Equine 25 (2009) 433–443
doi:10.1016/j.cveq.2009.07.005
0749-0739/09/$ – see front matter © 2009 Elsevier Inc. All rights reserved.

1. Equal Education Opportunity Act of 1974, which prohibited state denial of equal education by means of race, gender, color, or national origin
2. Since the 1980s, women have comprised most freshman admissions to college, and the gender gap has widened with time. Between 1970 and 2000, the number of women in postsecondary schools increased by 137% and the number in professional schools of all kinds increased by 853%. In 2004, 9.9 million women, compared with only 7.4 million men, were enrolled in accredited national colleges.[5]
3. Less economic reward in veterinary medicine as compared with other professions with a comparable educational debt load, suggesting the possibility that potential male applicants are attracted to other better paying professional career options
4. Advancements in chemical and other restraint methods allow safer handling of animals, and less body strength is required of veterinarians.
5. Enhanced societal recognition of the human-animal bond and the perception that women are somehow more compassionate
6. Mindset changes in the veterinary profession's acceptance or tolerance of part-time veterinarian workers, allowing women and men to choose career and family rather than one or the other

Some have also suggested that more women are attracted to small animal private practice than equine practice because they perceive it may be easier to obtain job-sharing part-time positions and to have more flexible hours, which, in turn, allow better time management of family responsibilities while having a career in veterinary medicine.[4]

As is discussed further in this article, flexible and innovative employment work schemes may work as well in equine practice as they do in other types of veterinary medical practice.

NATIONAL LABOR STATISTICS AND GENDER

It is helpful to examine the national status of wages, work hours, and other criteria of compensation first before discussing veterinary profession and equine practice trends. The overall observed gender compensation differences are a prelude to veterinary profession trends.

Earnings for women with college degrees have increased by approximately 33% since 1979 on an inflation-adjusted basis, whereas those of male college graduates have increased by 18%. Women working full-time in professional and related occupations earned $835 per week, the second highest paying job group after those in management, business, and financial operations occupations (median weekly earnings of $908 in 2007).[6]

Women are more likely than men to work in professional-related occupations but are not well represented in the higher paying professional job groups (computer and engineering fields) within this broad category. Professional women are more likely to work in education and health care fields (67% of female professionals vs 30% of male professionals). Median health care earnings were $920 per week as compared with earnings of significantly higher paying computer fields at $1229 per week.

Taking it one step further, according to the Bureau of Labor Statistics, when earnings of women and men were compared by the same area of expertise (by degree, degree level obtained, and age), approximately half of women earned approximately 87% of the earnings of men. In fact, professional medical degrees yielded women to be worth 86% of the earnings of men.[7]

The dental profession, which has historically been compared with the veterinary profession, exhibits the exact same discrepancy in salary. In 2007 to 2008, 44.6% of the predoctoral dental students and 44.5% of the graduates were female.[8] As with female physicians, female dentists make, on average, only 86% of the earnings of male dentists ($102,874 and $119,335, respectively).[9]

Median weekly earnings for married women and men were higher than those for unmarried workers. As a group, married workers tend to be older, suggesting they are more likely to be in prime earnings years. Among married workers of both genders, the earnings of those with children younger than the age of 18 years differed only slightly from the earnings of those without children. Among unmarried workers, women without children earned 14% more than those with children. The opposite was true among unmarried men: those with children earned 12% more than those with no children.

Among full-time workers, men were more likely than women to work longer hours per week. In 2007, 27% of men working full-time had work weeks of 41 hours or more, compared with 15% of female full-time workers. In contrast, women were three times as likely as men to work 35 to 39 hours per week (12% as opposed to 4%, respectively).

In the US labor force, women are more likely than men to work part-time, defined as fewer than 35 hours per week (25% of women vs 10% of men). These proportions have not changed much over time.

Information from the Monthly Labor Review, December 1999, helps to illuminate socioeconomic factors in the general working population.[10] Relative to unmarried women without children, married mothers and single mothers committed fewer hours to market work, but the differential had declined over the preceding 2 decades.

Further in this study, marriage has little effect on labor supply, although access to spousal income does exert a downward pressure on women's allocation of time to paid work. Although children exert less of a downward pressure on women's labor supply than they did in the late 1970s, the effect of preschool-aged children on working mothers' annual work hours is substantial.

ECONOMIC TRENDS IN VETERINARY COMPENSATION

Economic models of supply and demand apply to wages. The market for labor determines wages. The suppliers are individual doctors of veterinary medicine, who try to sell their labor for the highest price. Veterinary practices try to buy the type of labor they need at the lowest price. The equilibrium price for veterinary labor is the wage.

In the past decade, an increasing market for veterinary services in companion animal and equine practice has, in turn, led to increased competition for veterinary talent. Competition among many segments of career opportunity for graduates of veterinary colleges has led to increasing wages in general. It is likely that the profession's increasing recognition of competition for the best and brightest of college undergraduates has also had a positive impact on higher wages paid.

A significant gender compensation gap continues across the spectrum of professions, including veterinary medicine. Female veterinarians make approximately one-third less than their male counterparts, according to the 2008 AVMA Report on Veterinary Compensation based on the 2007 economic survey results. The good new seems to be that the gap is not growing for any particular demographic slice. The bad news is that starting salary differences of 6% continue to grow with time from graduation.

Examining differences at graduation, the annual *Journal of the American Veterinary Medical Association* survey of new graduates[11] states that the mean student debt among students who incurred student debt in 2008 was $121,006 for female graduates. The mean for male graduates was $115,059, however. The medians were $120,000 and $110,000 for women and men, respectively. In fact, a greater percentage of the female graduates (34.7%) graduated with a debt of $140,000 or more matched to 28.7% of the male graduates. In contrast to the rest of the data, more women (9.7%) graduated without debt compared with 8.7% of men. Therefore, with a higher overall student debt load and lower compensation, female veterinarians have a longer debt repayment period.

Male veterinarians should be as concerned about the gap as women are.[12] Depressed compensation implies that women may be producing less than a comparably experienced man working approximately the same hours. If that is the case, profitability for a given practice, or even many practices within a community, may be suppressed through lower average transaction charges. As repetitively published through various surveys and studies, lower professional earnings can discourage otherwise excellent candidates from seeking careers in veterinary medicine.

Several factors have been suggested but not definitively proved as affecting the apparent gender-based veterinary wage gap:

- Number of hours worked
- Level of experience
- Difference in negotiation skills of women as compared with men
- Satisfaction with pay[13]
- Gender discrimination

Gender discrimination seems to be disproved when comparing female veterinary practice owners with their male cohorts. In the Brakke study, female veterinarians with 14 years of experience received annual earnings of $56,214 as compared with men with 14 years of experience at $77,415. Furthermore, female owner compensation was 26% less than that of their male counterparts of equal stature.

According to the AVMA Economic Survey, the median 2007 professional income of all private practice veterinarians was $91,000, a 7.3% compounded increase over the 2005 median result of $79,000. For equine practitioners, there was no increase in the median income of $91,000 from 2005 to 2007. Mean equine practitioner income in 2005 was $128,302, and it was $131,195 in 2007.[14]

The 2008 AVMA report numbers indicate that new equine practitioners typically earn less than their small animal counterparts: $42,000 as compared with an average baseline starting salary of more than $65,000 for graduates entering exclusively small animal practice. The survey results show that after 5 years of practice, however, equine veterinarian income exceeds small animal doctors by more than $10,000 a year.

The 2008 AVMA survey reports continuing gaps between male and female veterinarians of all types, with a 34% gender difference for equine practitioners specifically, and without consideration of ownership. The income for female equine practitioners in 2007 increased 5.4% from that in 2005, compared with only a 2.3% increase for male equine practitioners in the 2-year period.

Examining equine practice owners only, female practitioners earn significantly less than their male counterparts. At the 50th and 90th percentiles, female owner compensation seemed to be approximately 60% that of male owners. The 75th percentile was especially dramatic, with female equine practitioner owners earning approximately 40% that of male cohort compensation.[15]

An earlier study[16] supports the AVMA 2007 Economic Survey results, showing statistical compensation differences based on gender. The purposes of the AVMA-Pfizer business practices study included measuring the effect of various management behaviors, attitudes, and actions (business practices) on income.

One study illustrated that female associates and owners receive less than male associates and owners when normalized for experience and hours worked. Another finding that was consistent with the results of the 1998 Brakke study suggested that female veterinarians who were highly satisfied with their incomes had substantially lower mean incomes than their male counterparts.[17]

The 2007 AAEP Lifestyle and Salary Survey[18] shows a large gender gap in reported income. Male respondents (n = 515) averaged $149,000. Female respondents (n = 541) averaged $81,820. These numbers do not correlate income with work schedule, hours worked, or production. Furthermore, the average age of male respondents was their mid-40s, whereas the average age of female respondents was their early 30s. When the 2007 AAEP study factored age into the computations, wage gaps grew significantly with increasing practitioner age.

The Brakke study found that women who scored higher in "business orientation" had higher mean incomes than did women who scored lower. Business orientation includes such behaviors as using financial concepts for practice management and establishing employee goals that align with practice goals. This suggests that a strong business orientation and higher salaries are directly correlated.

In this study, eight business practices were the leading predictors of higher personal incomes for both genders:

- Business orientation
- Frequency of financial data review
- Employee development
- Negotiating skill
- Client loyalty
- Leadership (motivating others)
- Client retention
- New client development

The AVMA-Pfizer study[12] and others have posed questions pertaining to gender compensation differences, as follows:

- Is the wage gap a result of adherence to traditional gender-based roles, such as women having more home responsibilities that reduce their professional performance (and value) as compared with men?
- Are women less productive because of those other commitments?
- Is satisfaction with a lower compensation amount partially a generational issue, in that a personal-professional life balance (job flexibility and reduced hours to pursue outside interests) is a valuable trade-off?
- Are employees who work for female owners compensated differently (perhaps better?), which accounts for the pay difference between male and female owners (ie, less profit remaining that would otherwise increase owner compensation)?
- Does owner compensation vary among professional practice owners who have different business acumen (not just years of experience)?
- Are student debt loads different between men and women, leading to greater urgency for repayment, reflected in higher compensation through negotiation and choice of employment positions or career options?

Studies indicate that male and female communication style differences may be a cause of gender-apparent compensation gaps.[19] Communication research about physicians and their patients suggests that female physicians "walk a fine line between exercising authority and appearing too authoritarian".[19] Lack of confidence and "soft" communication skills may lead to poorer client compliance with doctor recommendations, and resulting lower revenue. Lower revenue production leads to lower compensation.

Women can learn negotiation skills based on finding a win-win solution to doctor-client communication, which provides an opportunity to take care of the horse, the client, and the practice. Communication skill training may be an essential component of increasing all veterinarians' compensation.

PRACTICE OWNERSHIP OR PRACTICE ASSOCIATE?

The AVMA-Pfizer business practices study revealed that a smaller percentage of female associates (46%) expected to own veterinary practices as compared with male associates (53%). In this study, 17% of both genders had not yet decided on practice ownership.[17]

According to a 2007 Veterinary Economics Business Issues Study,[20] men still outnumber women by three to one in regard to practice ownership, even with some accounting for age discrepancies in the population of potential ownership candidates. By comparing the worth of female graduates over the decades with that of male graduates, female graduates of the 1990s and the new millennium are less likely to own practices compared with those who graduated before that time (28% and 7%, respectively).

Although the same trend is apparent for male ownership, the differences are not as steep. As a matter of fact, as the sampling pool became larger for the female veterinarians, the ownership values declined. The reverse was true for the men. Overall, men dominate the market, owning 70% of the practices, whereas women own 30%.

The 2007 AAEP Lifestyle and Salary Survey[18] queried owners and associates. Practice owners (79%) opined that it would be difficult to find a purchaser, and 45% may delay retiring as a result. Sixty-three percent of associates, interns, and residents said they would like to own a practice someday but were not certain of financial feasibility.

Some of the potential reasons suggested for the gender difference regarding ownership include the following:

- 80% of female associates cited "stress" as the largest disincentive to ownership[21]
- Limitations on personal life
- Long hours
- Financial risk

Highly personal values and opinions may lead to a decision not to own a practice.[22] Even so, it is important to recognize the potential high level of satisfaction that practice ownership provides, even with the sacrifices it requires.

The previously cited economic studies through the AVMA show that, in general, practice owners can expect to earn, on average, $40,000 per year more than associates. Compounded over many years of ownership, the additional earnings have significant value. The earlier that ownership is embarked on, the greater is the total return.

Furthermore, total remuneration can hinge on income returns associated with practice ownership that may not be clearly reflected in various economic surveys. For example, investment in associated practice real estate as an owner creates an additional income stream over and beyond that of the practice operating entity. Further, ownership conveys rights to the current income stream and to the appreciating value of the practice over time.

In addition to financial rewards, personal autonomy to make decisions can have important value to veterinarians, regardless of gender. A doctor of veterinary medicine is typically viewed as a community leader; therefore, functioning as a practice owner clearly enhances one's standing. For some, reputation and community standing as an owner can have substantial personal value and fulfillment.

Many veterinary associates who have moved to ownership roles did so because of the opportunity to mold a practice that fits with personal and professional goals. When changing to this role, veterinarians have greater control of their own professional future and economic well-being.

Anecdotally, a large number of female practice owners are seen across all practice types. Veterinary practice brokers have some of the best knowledge of current trends. Dr Richard Goebel's report on private survey results of brokers and transaction facilitators several years ago showed that approximately 53% of purchasers were men and 47% were women, and he senses little difference in 2008 to 2009 (R. Goebel, DVM, Simmons Veterinary Practice Sales and Appraisals, personal communication). His colleague, Dr David Gerber, says that 65% of recent practices sales in his northwest area were to female veterinarians, 29% were to male doctors, and 6% were to husband-wife teams (D. Gerber, DVM, Simmons Veterinary Practice Sales and Appraisals, personal communication).

Ownership opportunities for any veterinarian are expansive:

- Incremental buy-in to an existing practice
- Outright purchase of 100% of an existing practice
- Pairing up with another associate for shared purchase of 100% of an existing practice
- Practice startup

BELIEFS AND PERSONAL VALUE STRUCTURES

According to an article in *Veterinary Economics*,[23] a study published in the September 2008 issue of the *Journal of Applied Psychology* revealed that men who hold traditional views that women's primary responsibility is in the home earn approximately $8,500 more annually than those that are more egalitarian in their beliefs. Conversely, women with traditional views earn approximately $1,500 less than those with egalitarian beliefs.

This ideology is emulated in the veterinary graduating classes. According to the annual *Journal of the American Veterinary Medical Association* survey of new graduates,[11] 14.9% of male graduates have children, which is more than twice the number of female graduates with children (7.0%). In reality, more female graduates are single or have been divorced (63.6% and 4.3%, respectively) compared with the male graduates (59.8% and 1.7%, respectively).

In the 2007 AAEP Lifestyle and Salary Survey, 71% of female equine practitioners agreed that they had delayed or were postponing having children because of the impact on their career.

Working women may have personal value structures different from those of nonworking women.[24] Personal values drive decisions in which a person is faced with many alternative courses of action. According to references made within the article by Feather,[25] "values inform behavior standards, goals, one's assessment of how attractive outcomes, events, and objects are, and, in the end, one's motivation to do all sorts of things." The same researcher concludes that social value is more important to nonworking women than to working women and that economic and political values are more important to working women than to nonworking women.[25]

A popular explanation for women working is the need for money to make ends meet. Other factors have led to the sharp increase in married women's labor force participation since 1960, however, including education, increasing wage rate, declines in the male-female earnings gap, decline in gender discrimination, lower fertility, larger interval between marriage and the birth of the first child, use of birth control, household technology decreasing housework labor, and urbanization. Women increasingly perceive careers as sources of rewards that can be complementary to, rather than substitutable for, careers in the home.[26]

For some, the work-life balance seems to be a generational force as much as a gender issue. Some have stated that women value time off more than money and that vacation time and 4-day work weeks have greater value as work perks than does a high salary.[27]

Whether it is because they are predominantly women, or merely because they come from a generation with firm values regarding personal time, the new equine veterinarians who are now being managed have far different expectations than the old. Formerly, the desired equine veterinarian lifestyle was high stress in exchange for high salaries. The job, famous for being difficult and time-consuming, was pretty much guaranteed to be the center of one's life and one's top priority.

These new equine veterinarians come to the field with a new request, however: that their jobs allow them a greater measure of personal time. Small animal practices have taken the lead in management decisions to allow this to happen.

To attract and keep doctors, companion animal practices have offered shift work, job sharing, and special emergency clinics. Although, previously, these techniques seemed inapplicable to equine work, a wide variety of new solutions give this new generation what they desire: time.

Some practices have hired one emergency doctor to cover most evenings and weekends. The emergency veterinarian guarantees a more regular schedule for the other doctors, including a day that ends on time. The Marion Dupont Scott Equine Medical Center, a university hospital, and the Desert Pines Equine Center, a private practice, have used this strategy (N. A. White II, DVM, and L. Schur, DVM, personal communications, 2007).

With good communication, a strong record-keeping system, and associates who value their time off, client and case sharing is attainable. Excellent communication is vital when using multiple doctor personalities for patient coverage. It is important to reassure clients that with the changing of the guard, their horses' medical treatment is not going to suffer. In fact, a clear patient benefit is two sets of trained eyes monitoring the case.

For surgical practices, another successful job-sharing strategy uses two part-time surgeons. The emergency nature of most equine surgery often overloads the surgeon physically and mentally by continuous "on-call" responsibility. A two-surgeon practice can be an ideal solution for veterinarians raising families, by allowing each to devote specific days to family time without interruption.

Specialization has allowed some equine veterinarians to limit their work hours. With extra training in specialties like dentistry, acupuncture, or veterinary spinal manipulation therapy, which experience few or no emergencies, a doctor has more autonomy over his or her schedule. In Washington State, a dental specialist lives in the country but commutes to the Seattle area 2 weeks of the month to practice.

In Maryland, a boarded internal medicine specialist has an ambulatory consulting practice instead of being associated with one hospital. Through self-employment, a specialist can choose his or her hours and respective cases more freely.

None of these management practices work without a financially sound business model. Charging appropriately for services and collecting accounts receivable are vital to a financially stable veterinary practice with predictable cash flows to meet operating and capital requirements. Without strong business processes, veterinary practices of any kind cannot afford the correct number of staff, veterinarians, and technician hours to treat patients and serve clients unless shortcuts are taken. Shortcuts often lead to mistakes and malpractice situations. Practice owners must plan and sustain adequate profit for the long term so as to provide lifestyle schedules that allow veterinarians to pursue outside interests.

CHOICES, CHOICES, CHOICES

Regardless of gender and generation, doctors of veterinary medicine have many choices that ultimately affect career satisfaction, total compensation, lifestyle, and personal happiness. One woman's measuring stick is not necessarily another man's calibration of success. Success as a veterinarian has many different meanings and nuances.

Some life factors are outside our immediate control, such as gender, age, race, and family background. Yet, we can choose to control a large number of the factors that ultimately affect our personal parameters of economic and career satisfaction:

- Attitude
- Experience in leadership, work, and interpersonal roles
- Clinical experience and skill development
- Hours spent working as a veterinarian
- Practice community location, prosperity, and patient base opportunity
- Geographic region
- Business interest and acumen
- Personal financial management
- Age and reputation of the practice with which we choose to associate ourselves
- Practice culture and philosophy
- Whom we choose to be in business with
- Whom we choose to do business with
- Whom we choose to practice with

The crucial fact of our choice to join the veterinary profession is to commit to a life-long obligation of continual learning. From the moment we aspire to membership, we pledge to ever-increasing expansion of our knowledge (not only book knowledge but experiential knowledge).

The more we challenge ourselves with complex cases and with problems requiring scientific knowledge and communications skill, interlaced with intuition that comes from years of practice, the more valuable we become to our parallel communities of professional contribution, client service, and patient welfare.

Once embarked, any professional practices his or her profession. The quality of hours and quantity of challenging cases truly season a person, but perfection is rarely attained. The accumulation of abundant hours of practical experience compounds to economic value and personal satisfaction. Expecting high compensation by mere licensure is a poor tribute to veterinary medicine's rich tradition.

Each of us, man or woman, has different drivers of dedication to different goals. Many styles of practice serve those disparate and sometimes conflicting goals of financial well-being, patient care, and physical family presence. Each of us must titrate unique internal drivers of personal satisfaction and external forces to find a life's path that brings us to our best character.

ACKNOWLEDGMENTS

One of the authors (M.L.H.) acknowledges and extends appreciation for the research, editing, and advisory assistance of Erica R. Barron, senior veterinary student at The Ohio State University (class of 2009), and the research assistance of Jesse O. Bynum, an employee of the same author's veterinary consulting and accounting firm.

REFERENCES

1. Department of Labor, Women's Bureau. Women workers in ten war production areas and their postwar employment plans. Bulletin 209.
2. Holley S. Too many women in vet school or too few applicants? Cornell University Chronicle on Line; 2007.
3. Wright D. Animal attraction: women in contemporary veterinary medicine. Bryn Mawr College Science and Technology Newsletter.
4. Kitchner N. Wanted: country vets. Canadian Horse Annual 2009.
5. Leaving men behind: women go to college in ever-greater numbers. Available at: www.EducationPortal.com; Nov 13, 2007.
6. Highlights of women's earnings in 2007. US Department of Labor, US Bureau of Labor Statistics; 2008. Report 1008.
7. Hecker DE. Earnings of college graduates: women compared with men. Mon Labor Rev 1998;62–7.
8. 2007–08 survey of dental education, vol. 1. Academic programs, enrollment and graduates. Available at: www.ada.org/ada/prod/survey/faq.asp.
9. Salary survey report for job: dentist. Available at: www.payscale.com; 2009.
10. Cohen PN, Bianchi SM. Marriage, children, and women's employment: what do we know? Mon Labor Rev 1999;22.
11. Facts and figures, employment of female and male graduates of US veterinary medical schools and colleges, 2008. J Am Vet Med Assoc 2008;233(8).
12. Felsted KE, Volk JO. Why do women earn less? Vet Econ 2000;33.
13. Macejko C. AVMA salary survey shows DVMs earning more, dvm 360, Advanstar Communications, interview of Dr. Karen Felsted, CPA, CEO of the National Commission of Veterinary Economic Issues.
14. Income of US Veterinarians, 2007. J Am Vet Med Assoc 2009;234(6).
15. 2007 AVMA Economic survey results presented by Webinar on AVMA Web site. 2009.
16. AVMA-Pfizer Business Practices Study. January 10, 2005.
17. Volk JO, et al. Executive summary of the AVMA-Pfizer business practices study. J Am Vet Med Assoc 2005;226:212–8.
18. Preston-Osborne marketing communications and research. Lexington (KY).
19. Miller J. Are women tough enough? Vet Econ 2008;6(49).
20. Gender shift: women are less likely to own a practice, even when you account for age. Vet Econ 2008.
21. 2007 Veterinary Economics Business Issues Study.
22. King D. What are the benefits of owning a practice? Available at: www.SimmonsInc.com.

23. Gender pay gap is all in the mind and very real. Vet Econ 2008.
24. Jalilvand M. Married women, work, and values. Mon Labor Rev 2000;26.
25. Feather NT. Values, valences, and choice: the influence of values on the perceived attractiveness and choice of alternative. J Pers Soc Psychol 1995;1135–51.
26. Mott FL, Shapior D. Complementarity of work and fertility among young American mothers. J Popul Stud 1983;239–52.
27. Fiala J. Women rock gender balance in profession, dvm360, advanstar, March 3, 2003 interview comments of Tracy Dowdy, a consultant with Brakke Consulting, Inc.

The Transition from Veterinary School to Equine Practice

Katherine S. Garrett, DVM

KEYWORDS

• Equine • Internship • Practice • Education
• Transition • Veterinary • Lifestyle

The information in this article was gathered through informal conversations with many practitioners at different stages of their career. Although there are few facts and figures, this work is a compilation of information that veterinarians wish they had known when they graduated from veterinary school, advice they have received or have given, and personal experiences. There are not clear-cut answers to most questions confronting new graduates; thus, this should be taken as friendly advice from those who have been there.

THE REAL WORLD

Moving from the life of a student to the life of a professional is exciting but can be difficult and unsettling at times. Although some new graduates may have come to veterinary medicine as a second career, many new graduates are entering a profession for the first time. Recent graduates are expert students, having spent approximately 20 years undergoing formal education. More recently, they have learned to succeed as veterinary students. The transition from veterinary school to practice, wherein a whole new set of skills is necessary for success, can be a huge challenge. Put another way, new graduates know a lot of information, but they may not know how to apply their knowledge to managing actual clinical cases or performing technical skills adeptly. Veterinary students are essentially sheltered from real responsibility and consequences of poor decisions. Although most veterinary students eagerly await the day they can make the decisions, the sudden assumption of responsibility after graduation can be unnerving.

The overall pace of the workday is much faster in private practice than in a university setting. The importance of efficiency cannot be stressed enough. Inefficiency as a student generally only affects one person. In practice, inefficiency at the first appointment has a cascading effect through the day and also affects clients, patients,

---

Department of Diagnostic Imaging, Rood and Riddle Equine Hospital, 2150 Georgetown Road, PO Box 12070, Lexington, KY 40580, USA
E-mail address: kgarrett@roodandriddle.com

Vet Clin Equine 25 (2009) 445–454
doi:10.1016/j.cveq.2009.07.002
0749-0739/09/$ – see front matter © 2009 Elsevier Inc. All rights reserved.

technicians, and the bottom line. Not only is the time commitment as a practicing veterinarian greater than the time commitment as a student, but the schedule is often more unpredictable. A well-planned day can be thrown into disarray with the need to attend to an emergency. Many aspects of equine practice (eg, breeding, foaling, competition) are seasonal, leading to busier times of the year interposed with slower times.

There are other personal factors contributing to this feeling of flux. Many graduates move to new places, where they may know no one. Creating a network of friends in an unfamiliar city is more difficult than making friends in an educational setting, where many classmates have also moved to a new place and are looking for new friends. Most equine practices are not in urban centers with high concentrations of young professionals, complicating efforts to expand one's social network. Additional life changes, such as recent marriage or birth of children, can add to the list of stressors.

FINDING AN INTERNSHIP

Many recent graduates choose to spend their first year of practice in the more struc-tured educational environment provided by an internship. An internship is a postgrad-uate year spent practicing under the supervision of more experienced practitioners. Ideally, an internship serves as a bridge between the role of a veterinary student with limited or no responsibility and the role of an associate with significant primary case responsibility and the ability to handle it. In the opinion of the author and of those practitioners interviewed, an internship is invaluable.

The number of equine private practice internships has grown tremendously over the past 10 years, with nearly 150 practices listed in the Avenues section of the American Association of Equine Practitioners (AAEP) Web site.[1] Many practices offer multiple positions. The large percentage of new graduates in equine practice seeking an intern-ship may be in response to the recognition that it is difficult to graduate from veterinary school and immediately be competent enough to step into the role of an associate in an equine practice. This may be attributable to the emphasis on small animal medicine in veterinary school. A study of veterinary students showed that improvements in clin-ical reasoning after a year of clinical rotations were greater in situations involving small animals than in those involving large animals, regardless of the chosen clinical track of the student.[2]

Also, a new graduate entering a small animal group practice as an associate is in an environment in which seeking advice from a colleague is logistically simple; a more experienced colleague is often in the next room. Most equine practices offering asso-ciate positions to new graduates are ambulatory practices. Doctors typically travel solo or with a technician; thus, seeking advice can be more challenging. A telephone call may be sufficient to check a drug choice but may be inadequate when one is faced with a challenging lameness case or ophthalmic problem.

Additionally, equine veterinarians often examine a case and formulate a plan with the owner present. Because many horse owners are well educated about their animals, this adds another layer of pressure for a new graduate. The importance of the relationship between a veterinarian and the client cannot be underestimated. Employers cited client interaction skills as the most important interpersonal skill set when hiring new graduate veterinarians.[3] After completing an internship, a recent graduate is more competent in diagnosis and treatment, having seen many cases with experienced guidance. This competence leads to increased confidence, trans-lating into greater client comfort and satisfaction. An internship also provides a graduate with a group of more experienced veterinarians on whom to rely for assistance in the future.

There are as many types of internships as there are internship programs. The options range from university internships, to small ambulatory practice internships, to large hospital-based programs. The amount of supervision, didactic instruction, primary case responsibility, and emergency duty varies among programs. It is essential to choose a program that is a good fit for a specific individual, and no one program is perfect. Some general characteristics of high-quality internship programs include adequate supervision, the ability to see a wide variety of cases and treatment options, and a commitment on the part of the practice to education and mentoring. Externships are an excellent way to be exposed to private practice and to investigate possible internship opportunities.

When considering postgraduate training, bear in mind that an internship, by its definition, involves supervision and training. "Intern" is not a synonym for "low-paid associate." Nevertheless, an internship is not a glamorous job and does occasionally involve performing seemingly mundane tasks. With that said, the intern must take responsibility for his or her education. The balance between appropriately taking the initiative and overstepping one's bounds can be delicate. Rather than blindly following directions, he or she should take the time to think through the rationale for the treatment plan in general and as applied to a specific individual, bearing in mind that there are many ways to manage a case successfully.

FINDING A JOB

Before seeking employment, it is wise to consider a wide variety of factors. These may include the type and size of the practice; geographic considerations (eg, proximity to friends, family, urban areas, outdoor activities); opportunities for continued mentorship; possibilities for practice ownership; and the types, breeds, and uses of the horses in the practice. This list can help to narrow down a long list of practices to a group that is more manageable. This exercise may also help to focus one's attention on factors that are nonnegotiable and areas on which compromise is possible. This intangible balance is different for every individual, and it is of paramount importance to be honest with one's self about this priority list and to re-evaluate it periodically. Seeking out advice from a variety of sources can be helpful. These may include more experienced veterinarians, family members, or friends. Each group has a unique perspective and can provide different food for thought. In the end, however, the decision must be one's own. It may help to remember that one's first job does not have to be the ultimate job.

Sorting through employment listings to find a job for the long term after an internship or immediately after graduation can be difficult. Potential positions may be formally listed in journals or on Web sites, such as that of the AAEP. Individual practices may post advertisements on their own Web sites or seek out potential associates informally through conversations with colleagues about their current interns or students. Information about vacancies may be spread simply through word of mouth; thus, the involvement of mentors can be valuable. In some cases, it may be appropriate to approach a practice that is not actively advertising.

Personal or telephone interviews give the applicant and the practice an opportunity to discuss concrete matters, such as compensation, schedule, and responsibilities. The practice philosophy can be discussed, but there is little substitute for an on-site visit to gain a first-hand impression of the practice culture and style and the personalities involved. The members of the practice and the applicant should be fully invested in these conversations so as to make an informed decision, because areas of potential conflict may not be immediately obvious on the surface.

It is important to recognize that some of the factors contributing to success in practice may be different than those contributing to success in veterinary school. Although achieving academic success largely relies on retention of a large body of information, good study habits, and excellent performance during formal examinations, success in practice requires these skills in addition to working well with colleagues and staff, effective communication, sound decision making, management of time, and a myriad of other skills not emphasized in most veterinary curricula.[4] When evaluating potential new associates, practice owners cited interpersonal skills as the most important factor, with an interview and practice visit as the best way to assess these intangible traits.[3]

Even with an exhaustive interview process and multiple visits, the match between the practice and a newly hired associate sometimes turns out not be a good fit for all involved for any number of reasons. Although no one likes to be in these situations, they do happen. In these cases, it is important for both parties to be honest and realize that a change may need to be made.

FINANCIAL CONSIDERATIONS

As the debt load incurred during undergraduate and veterinary studies increases,[5] strategies for managing this burden are important. During school, pursuing scholarships or part-time employment can assist with reducing the amount owed. Consultation with a financial planner may uncover avenues to manage debt incurred for education and personally. Deferral of loans may be an option in some situations. Employers should realize that the current debt load is significantly larger than what they may have experienced when they graduated from veterinary school, and a frank conversation between the potential associate and employer may be needed.

Once a salary has been finalized, it may be prudent for a recent graduate to establish a budget to determine realistically what the estimated take-home pay per month is going to be. This can help one to map out projected expenses for housing, food, loan payments, utility bills, car payments, and entertainment, for example. It is easier to plan ahead to make sure that one is not overextended financially and makes appropriate choices than to realize too late that one's income is not covering one's expenses.

A recent meta-analysis of new graduates' financial situations has reported that the starting salary of equine practitioners is significantly lower than that of veterinarians in other types of practice, with the highest debt-to-starting salary ratio.[5] One of the likely reasons for the discrepancy during the first year after graduation is the high percentage of graduates pursing equine practice who choose to complete an internship compared with the lower percentage of graduates entering small animal practice who complete an internship. The mean and median incomes of equine practitioners overall are greater than those of any other practice type,[6] suggesting that over time, the salaries of equine practitioners outstrip those of small animal practitioners.

Although an internship typically has a lower salary than an associate's position, equine private practitioners who have completed an internship eventually earn more than their colleagues who have not completed an internship.[7] Taking a long-term view of lifetime earnings paints a more complete picture on which to base a decision. One way to value an investment in education is to realize that salary is dictated by the amount of revenue created for the practice. By becoming more efficient and skilled (through an internship, a residency, or other advanced educational opportunities), one can work less time for the same revenue and salary or can work the same amount of time for an increased revenue and salary.

BALANCING PERSONAL AND PROFESSIONAL LIVES

The stereotypical equine practitioner works long hours for low pay, has minimal time off, is constantly available, and has little time for family. Although there are practitioners with this lifestyle, it is certainly not the only model. Different people have different priorities for a myriad of reasons. Some people prefer a flexible or part-time schedule over large financial rewards, whereas others prize monetary compensation more highly. The important thing is to realize what one's own priorities are and to find employment that serves these goals, realizing that compromises have to be made. There are many people who would like flexible hours, excellent benefits, a high salary, no emergency duty, a practice in a specific geographic area, and the ability to see cases only in certain subject areas. That scenario is unrealistic in most (if not all) instances, however. Sacrifices have to be made in some areas. In particular, long hours are fairly typical for new graduates entering equine practice, and the 4-day work week is the exception rather than the norm. The specific choices a person makes are obviously unique to his or her situation, but it is naive to believe that nothing has to be compromised. When applying for employment and assessing one's career path, these factors must be borne in mind.

One aspect of equine practice that complicates scheduling is the relative nonexistence of emergency clinics. Most small animal practices do not accept after-hours or weekend emergencies and refer their clients to a local emergency clinic. This scenario is extremely rare in equine practice. As a result, someone has to be available to attend to these patients. Practices vary in how emergencies are handled; some rotate emergency duty among doctors within the practice, and some form partnerships with practices in the same area and rotate emergency duty among practices, with many additional models in existence. Whatever the arrangement, it is extremely unlikely that a new graduate can entirely avoid emergency work; in many cases, he or she may perform more emergency work than more senior members of the practice. If a new graduate is saddled with an unreasonable proportion of the emergency duty; however, resentment and dissatisfaction are likely to build; thus, a balance must be struck.

Although inconvenient, going on emergency calls can be a valuable learning experience. Prompt, professional, and courteous service on an emergency basis may encourage clients to be more accepting of the "new vet" when they are scheduling elective procedures later and have their choice of doctors. Discussion of unusual or difficult cases fosters communication among members of the practice, building rapport and allowing a new graduate to draw on the valuable bank of knowledge available from more experienced practitioners.

Considerable attention has been paid to the "generation gap" between what has been termed the *Boomer Generation* (born in 1946-1964) and *Generations X* (born in 1965–1978) and *Y* (born in 1978–2000).[8] These concerns are not limited to equine practice or veterinary medicine; they have been topics of discussion in many professions, including the field of human medicine.[9] As a generalization, the boomers value total dedication to work, whereas Generations X and Y prioritize a balance between work and personal life.[8,9] One writer summarized that "Gen Y...thinks Gen X...is a bunch of whiners. Gen X sees Gen Y as arrogant and entitled. And everyone thinks the Baby Boomers...are self-absorbed workaholics".[10] Although no one person can be reduced to a stereotype and exceptions to the rule are enormously common, there may be a grain of truth in these thoughts that bears consideration.

These differences have been considered in equine practice specifically. In a 2007 survey of AAEP members, 78% of respondents older than the age of 50 years agreed with the statement "Younger practitioners are not as committed to the profession of equine medicine as were those who came before them," whereas 85% of respondents younger than the age of 40 years agreed that "Older practitioners don't respect younger practitioners' desire to strike a better work/personal life balance".[7] Perhaps it is more helpful to attempt to communicate openly to understand and respect others' values and motivations to help bridge this gap, recognizing that there is no one "right way." Although one should be true to one's priorities regarding a work-life balance, it is important to be mindful that for at least the next decade, most employers are members of the Boomer Generation and a new associate may need to prove that he or she can and intends to work hard before asserting priorities.

Because equine practice is physically and mentally demanding, taking care of one's self increases longevity in the profession. Although it is important to learn from one's mistakes, dwelling on them longer than necessary is counterproductive and stress needs to be managed appropriately. This can include taking time to remember the reasons for choosing this career path instead of constantly being bogged down in the minutia. One aspect of practice that can be particularly enjoyable is sharing in the success of patients in the show ring, on the racetrack, as a trail horse, or as a 4-H project. Having outside interests helps to maintain perspective and prevent burnout.

Although often taken for granted, staying physically fit and eating a healthy diet help to prevent injuries and contribute to more rapid healing if injuries do occur. Practicing proper radiation safety and appropriate restraint should be routine, but there is always a temptation to slip into bad habits, and the veterinarian sets the example for clients, technicians, and students.

IT'S ALL ON THE TEST

It is impossible to cover the entire body of knowledge that comprises veterinary medicine of all species in 4 years of veterinary school. Additionally, there are new techniques and areas developed constantly. For example, molecular biology and associated gene therapies were not taught 30 years ago, but they are now considered to be important emerging areas. As a result of the enlarging knowledge base, some areas necessarily receive less coverage.

Our equine patients are unaware of this massive body of knowledge, however, and their owners require quality care for their animals. In a way, everything is on the test, not just what was covered in lectures or was tested on the examination. We are all responsible for all the material in some sense. That being said, no one is an expert on every subject; this includes realizing one's limitations and knowing when and how to seek additional help. Throughout their careers, all practitioners are confronted with unusual clinical presentations or a case that is not routine. Although this is one of the most exciting and intellectually challenging facets of veterinary medicine, it can require a change in perspective from veterinary school.

This means that one's educational mindset needs to mature from trying to memorize facts to becoming a critical clinical thinker. Having an answer quickly is not necessarily the goal; the most important thing is the thought process and reasoning behind the decision. This allows evaluation of successes and failures so as to learn from experience. In addition to honing problem-solving skills, it is important to learn how to build on the educational base from veterinary school. This can take many forms, from keeping abreast of current literature, to doing additional research on a challenging case, to being willing to listen to more seasoned colleagues' experience with a particular disorder.

Although seemingly basic, physical examination skills cannot be overemphasized. We are fortunate to live in an era with advanced diagnostic equipment available, but there is no substitute for a thorough physical examination. Physical examination is generally noninvasive, inexpensive, and available to every practitioner. Clients value a veterinarian who is able to make a reasonable diagnosis in a cost-effective manner and uses diagnostic tests appropriately but not excessively. Performing a complete examination of every case, even if the appointment is only for a simple injection, teaches a new graduate the wide variety of findings that can still be considered "normal." It can be difficult to determine when a true abnormality exists without a firm grasp of what is normal, and this can only be gained through experience with large numbers of cases.

MENTORSHIP

One of the most frequently cited pieces of advice given to new graduates is to find a mentor. It seems simple, but it can be much more difficult in reality, because relationships such as these take time to nurture and mature. One study showed that most mentors in veterinary medicine are employers and that the most important attributes from the mentee's perspective are trust, support, and "accepting the protégé as a competent professional".[11] Getting involved in professional organizations can be a way in which to find mentors outside one's own practice and eventually to serve as a mentor to others. The AAEP, state veterinary medical associations, and breed- or discipline-specific organizations are all good places to start. Former professors often become mentors as well. The relationship becomes mutually beneficial as new graduates seek advice, professors keep abreast of developments in private practice, and former students often become referring veterinarians. Effective mentoring relationships are often not formal but grow slowly and change over time. Shared values and working styles also contribute to the success of these relationships, and veterinarians who were mentored reported more professional success as compared with those who were not mentored.[11]

By the same token, realize that you may be a mentor to veterinary students or preveterinary students. A younger veterinarian may be more approachable to a veterinary student and have similar concerns and questions while being able to bridge the gap between students and older practitioners. Treat students with respect because they are future veterinarians and colleagues and remember the importance of mentorship in your own career. A conversation about the rewards and challenges of equine medicine may be more pivotal in a student's career choice than you realize.

SKILLS YOU CAN OFFER

Although new graduates do not have the experience that older practitioners do, they do tend to have exposure to the latest technology gained from veterinary school or an internship. It is much easier to have a person on the staff who is comfortable with the equipment and who can troubleshoot common problems than to have to call technical support late at night or on a weekend and explain a confusing error message over the telephone. Additionally, younger veterinarians may be more computer-savvy in general, bringing additional nonmedical skills with them, such as the ability to create or maintain a practice Web site. They may be able to ease a transition to digital medical records for older practitioners, being able to synthesize their medical knowledge with technical expertise.

New graduates have also been exposed to the latest research and treatments being used at university hospitals. They may bring a fresh perspective on a case workup or a new technique. The experience of older practitioners can be combined with the recent education of a new graduate. There are additional intangible benefits that a recent graduate may bring, including enthusiasm and the energy to work hard.

CREATING A NICHE

Although a broad foundation on which to draw is invaluable, some areas of practice are inevitably more interesting than others. A new graduate should find aspects of equine medicine that are enjoyable and spend time learning more about them. Ideally, the areas that interest the new associate are areas in which the practice would benefit from additional expertise. In other cases, these areas are incongruous. Bear in mind that developing competence in an area that is not engaging solely for the sake of the practice's needs may not be a good long-term strategy. It is difficult to devote the amount of time and practice necessary to master a skill if the subject matter is not interesting. Often, the result is procrastination and no increase in skill level, when the time could have been devoted to developing a skill that can be retained and used throughout a career.

Finding the aspects of medicine that are particularly interesting and then developing competency in these areas is the most effective way to create a niche in a practice. At times, the learning process can be frustrating, difficult, and time-consuming, but skills improve with the investment of self-directed effort. Gaining expertise in a particular area contributes to long-term job satisfaction and prevents burnout, because ongoing challenges keep the job interesting. Over time, as skill level and client demand increase, the percentage of one's time spent working in a niche increases, improving skills further.

Although bringing new services to the practice may involve some initial expense on the practice's part (eg, continuing education fees, purchase of equipment), there are obvious longer term benefits. Services that previously were referred to other practices or university hospitals can be kept within the practice, and new clients may be attracted. This not only makes sense from a financial standpoint but from client satisfaction and patient care perspectives. Greater continuity of care is achieved, and follow-up examinations or treatments can be completed more easily without potential travel for the client.

PROFESSIONALISM

When meeting a new associate or intern, the office staff, technicians, other veterinarians, and clients are operating with limited knowledge; thus, first impressions are important. Being on time, prepared, neat, and professionally attired can go a long way in establishing the trust essential in one's professional relationships. In general, veterinary clinics are still fairly conservative places of business.

Willingness to be a team player and a good colleague is invaluable. Although it is unnecessary to be best friends with everyone in the practice, an ability to get along and work with people on a professional level is vital. Technicians and office staff deserve to be treated with respect at all times but especially when clients are present. In return, they can often make initially hesitant clients with whom they have a rapport more accepting of a new doctor.

Excellent communication skills cannot be overemphasized. The goal is effective communication with peers, academicians, employers, technical and office staff, owners, and grooms without alienating or insulting any of them. Clients desire and deserve to be informed about results of diagnostic tests and the treatment plan for their horses. Equine medicine is ultimately a service business; thus, being an asset to the practice by providing good customer service is paramount.

If one is unsure of a diagnosis or appropriate treatment in a case, clients generally seem to appreciate an honest approach and a willingness to seek help when necessary as opposed to false confidence. No one knows everything, and it is often easier and results in a better outcome to ask for help sooner rather than later. There are multiple resources available (eg, books, notes, colleagues, clinicians at universities or local referral practices), and one should not be shy about using them. If better facilities, availability of equipment, or additional expertise would benefit the horse, it is always appropriate to suggest referral as an option to a client. Referral of a case is not a sign of failure.

Ethical issues, by their very nature, are often not easy to handle. The decisions one makes early in one's career often set the tone for a lifetime of practice. New veterinarians may be looked at as "easy targets" by the few unscrupulous clients who might take advantage of the situation. One needs to set one's own moral compass and stand by it, which can be difficult, because there can be competing desires to serve the client, please one's employer, and to do the ethical thing. Choosing a practice with a philosophy and morals consistent with your own can help to reduce these tensions.

SUMMARY

Finally, it is worth mentioning a few words of advice that were common threads in the conversations with all the practitioners interviewed. Be willing to do (almost) anything that is asked of you. Enthusiasm, a positive attitude, and a strong work ethic can take you far and make up for a lack of experience. Be proactive in educating yourself, and do not expect to be spoon-fed information. Take responsibility for yourself and your actions. Most importantly, provide excellent patient care.

Equine practice is an incredibly rewarding career. The first few years after graduation could be considered the most important in one's practice lifetime. Habits are formed and standards are set early. Although it can be daunting and exhausting, investing in your career by working hard, continually challenging yourself, and taking advantage of additional educational opportunities (formal and informal) can pay great dividends later in your career. That being said, it is vital to know your own priorities, professional goals, and personal values and aspirations so as to make decisions that lead to fulfillment.

REFERENCES

1. American Association of Equine Practitioners. Avenues. Available at: http://www.aaep.org/avenues_result.php?practicename=&state=&deadline=&type=INTERNSHIP&btnSearch=SEARCH. Accessed February 14, 2009.
2. Farnsworth CC, Herman JD, Osterstock JB, et al. Assessment of clinical reasoning skills in veterinary students prior to and after the clinical year of training. J Am Vet Med Assoc 2008;233:879–82.
3. Heath TJ, Mills JN. Criteria used by employers to select new graduate employees. Aust Vet J 2000;78:312–6.
4. Lewis RE, Klausner JS. Nontechnical competencies underlying career success as a veterinarian. J Am Vet Med Assoc 2003;222:1690–6.

5. Chieffo C, Kelly AM, Ferguson J. Trends in gender, employment, salary, and debt of graduates of US veterinary medical schools and colleges. J Am Vet Med Assoc 2008;233:910–7.

6. Shepherd AJ. Income of US veterinarians, 2005. J Am Vet Med Assoc 2007;231: 872–4.

7. Preston-Osborne. A confidential lifestyles and salary survey. American Association of Equine Practitioners, Lexington (KY); 2008.

8. Stefaniak A, Vetter C. Black hole or window of opportunity? Understanding the generation gap in today's workplace. Center for Public Policy and Administration, The University of Utah, Salt Lake City. 2007. Available at: http://www.cppa.utah.edu/publications/workforce/Generations.pdf. Accessed February 15, 2009.

9. Smith LG. Medical professionalism and the generation gap. Am J Med 2005;118: 439–42.

10. Gelston S. Gen Y, Gen X, and the baby boomers: workplace generation wars. CIO. 2009. Available at: http://www.cio.com.au/article/205772/gen_y_gen_x_baby_boomers_workplace_generation_wars?pp=1. Accessed February 16, 2009.

11. Niehoff BP, Chenoweth P, Rutti R. Mentoring within the veterinary medical profession: veterinarians' experiences as protégés in mentoring relationships. J Vet Med Educ 2005;32:264–71.

Ethics in Equine Practice Economics

Terry D. Swanson, DVM

KEYWORDS

• Equine • Ethics • Morals • Leadership • Core values

Professional ethics is the "virtually infallible standard" (Dr Jim Coffman, American Association of Equine Practitioners [AAEP] presidential address, 1986[1]) for our actions as equine veterinarians. Our ethical standards define how we relate to the horse, to the client, to fellow veterinarians, to employees, and to society. Our professional ethics are significantly influenced by our personal morals. Therefore, it is difficult to separate professional ethics from personal ethics or morals. However, there are specific principles set down for guidelines of our actions within our profession. Webster[2] defines ethical as conformity with a code of moral principles of a particular profession. Morals, as defined by Webster[2], are principles or standards with respect to right or wrong in conduct.

The AAEP has an ethical code that, with addendums, supports the code of the American Veterinary Medical Association. This code spells out the specific actions we, as professionals, should take to function in a manner to benefit our horses and society. As with any "legislation," there is room for interpretation. For members of the AAEP, these conflicts are resolved by the Peer Review Committee on Professional Conduct and Ethics.

Because ethics are an "ideal code of moral principles," we need to look also at our individual moral principles. For many reasons, each individual has his or her own template of moral principles. In essence, we all come from a different place, even if slight, with regard to moral principles. Therefore, although most veterinarians have like-minded principles, there is still room for varying interpretation of specific circumstances. Then, there are others who come from the wider ends of the bell curve, which broadens the outlook on a situation. These situations require more review, interpretation, discussion, and compromise to reach a consensus.

Please note that any actions outside the letter of the law are beyond this discussion of ethics.

Our individual moral principle template is set to some degree when we arrive in society as a newborn. Then, it is shaped by many external forces as we mature and interact within our society. The most obvious of these forces is probably the influence of parents and other family members. There are also specific individuals at different

Littleton Equine Medical Center, 8025 South Santa Fe Drive, Littleton, CO 80120, USA
E-mail address: doctds@msn.com

Vet Clin Equine 25 (2009) 455–461
doi:10.1016/j.cveq.2009.07.009
0749-0739/09/$ – see front matter © 2009 Elsevier Inc. All rights reserved.

stages of our life, grade school, high school, and college who we choose to admire as mentors. This is no doubt an extremely influential time in our moral development and a benchmark setting. Therefore, for healthy development, it is important that we be exposed to positive circumstances during this time. In contrast to a positive mentor, there can also be individuals who have a negative impact on our moral character. This may be a mentor who betrays the moral fiber to which we have subscribed, such as a teacher who talks the high road, but we discover that he or she behaves differently in real life. We can be enamored by the apparent success of an individual who operates in an immoral fashion, like a friend who gets good grades by cheating. These experiences can have a negative influence on our own development. Hopefully, more often than not, these instances strengthen our convictions. Certainly, we must learn to measure other people and understand at what level of moral principle they function. These circumstances can be true at all stages of our life; however, recognizably, we are less influenced as we mature and have benchmarked our own moral principles.

Influences in veterinary school have an impact on our moral principles at the professional level, while giving us opportunity to practice our own principles. Once out of veterinary school, our professional colleagues and mentors again help to shape and validate our moral standards, making it important to evaluate and choose with care and discernment the veterinarians with whom we practice. Likewise, this applies to the clients we prefer to serve. We can survive only so long in an environment that is contrary to our moral principles. We may become discontent, or worse, our morals may be devalued.

We enjoy one of the most credible of all professions. As individuals, we need to keep strong personal and professional moral standards for the sake of our profession and its influence on society. This is especially true in today's world, wherein many business and political people are rewarded by only taking care of themselves to the detriment of others. Some are doing this in such an excessive fashion that it is hard to comprehend.

In the course of daily life and practice, our values are challenged. Therefore, it is important that we have given serious thought to our personal ethics and moral principles beforehand. We need to know where we each come from as individuals and why. We must have conviction that right is right and to do the right thing even or especially when it is difficult. The personal satisfaction of taking the high road, no matter how difficult, is reward, in addition to the earned support of other principled professionals. This ratifies our convictions in managing future challenges and increases future credibility.

ETHICAL CHALLENGES

Clients can request certain procedures that are not ethical, such as altering a horse's appearance with surgery by removing a white spot from a horse's skin. The request can be out of ignorance or true malice. To change the appearance of a breeding horse is a form of deceit. If the client is ignorant of his or her responsibilities as a horse owner, the veterinarian can usually correct his or her thoughts with some good educational discussions. If the request is intentionally unethical, education can fall on deaf ears. This client could be willing to find someone else to perform the procedure, but it is still important to explain to the client why the procedure is unethical.

Newly graduated veterinarians and established veterinarians are subject to requests from unethical clients. First, the new veterinarian may be "tried" to see if he or she honors such a request. Second, as a result of long-term client relationships, established veterinarians can be asked to perform unethical procedures because of past client loyalty, particularly if the client has fallen on hard financial times.

Client confidentiality regarding his or her horse and its conditions can often be difficult to maintain in equine practice. The local equine community is small in terms of the numbers of people. They often know what has occurred with a friend's or acquaintance's horse and, from curiosity, request information about its well-being. Although the request can be innocent, we must remember that the information is confidential and privileged to the owner. Again, this is usually a matter of client education delivered with sensitivity.

The author would like to relate a personal anecdote regarding client confidentiality. While making country calls, he encountered the high-school son of a regular client. They had a general discussion about horses and the weather. As the author began to leave, the boy inquired where he was going. The author was sure that the boy was asking the question out of curiosity about his activities as an equine veterinarian and not to pry into another horseman's business. To maintain confidentiality for the neighboring client, however, the author replied "down the road." The boy repeated the question, and the author repeated his answer; then, with a quizzical grin, the boy said goodbye. Many years later, the same young man had become a professional horse trainer. On a visit to his barn, he reminded the author of the incident years before, and the author acknowledged that he remembered. Then, the young man said, "I get it."

Prepurchase examination results are another important area of client confidentiality. The information gleaned is owned solely by the person requesting and paying for the examination. This becomes more of a conflict if the buyer does not purchase the horse. Then, there are other potential buyers who would like the examination results. These data can only be released if the first buyer agrees. If the seller is absent during the examination, most buyers would release the results to the seller. This would be a common courtesy, but it is only implied and must be validated by the first buyer.

Upholding the rules of a breed registry or a racing jurisdiction is an important ethical process. We are to presume that these rules or regulations are for the benefit of the horse. If there is a question about the nature of a rule or regulation, we must take our concerns to the proper authorities and provide accurate scientific reasoning for our opinion.

Overuse of medication in an attempt to influence performance is unethical, especially if the welfare of the horse is affected. An example would be the use of several anti-inflammatory medications concurrently, or "stacking" of these medications.

In cases of referral or second opinion, our actions and discussions should be considerate to the initial examining veterinarian. We have no way to know exactly the status of the horse as it was presented to him or her. Additionally, the owner's attitude and needs could have been different at that time. An example is a colic case; initially, the owner said surgery was not a viable option, and the veterinarian used medications that would not ordinarily be used on a presurgical case. When the horse did not respond to therapy, the owner decided to seek a second opinion. After counsel with the referral veterinarian, the owner elected to have surgery on his horse. The referral veterinarian should not criticize the examining veterinarian in this circumstance for administering the initial medication.

There are circumstances in which a client changes his or her story when seeing a second veterinarian for the same problem. The reason may be guilt for inattention to the problem initially or for his or her lack of attention after the initial treatment. The second veterinarian must choose words wisely pending all the details. The reason may be a legitimate loss of trust in the first veterinarian; however, again, the second veterinarian must be careful with his or her words. It is reasonable to ask to visit with the first veterinarian to get the facts straight. If there is a genuine difference in how the horse should be treated, direct communication between the veterinarians should be a healthy resolution.

Within equine practice, it is ethically important that veterinarians respect the relationship each client has with fellow veterinarians. For whatever reason makes it necessary, caring for the horse of a colleague's regular client is professionally important, but courting that client for your own gain would not be morally correct. Being openly critical of another veterinarian's judgment or methods in the presence of the client would be unethical unless there is an immediate danger to the horse, owner, or staff.

Greed is likely the most significant reason for a well-intentioned veterinarian to lose track of his or her moral responsibilities. This may be in response to personal economic stresses, family pressures, or the need to achieve certain goals that he or she feels are slipping away. The veterinarian may simply be looking for a short cut.

Apathy and complacency can also undermine the leadership of a practice when certain goals have been achieved and the drive for healthy control of the practice slips away.

The ethical code for equine veterinarians can be reviewed in more detail in the AAEP Resource Guide and Membership Directory.[3] Questions of ethical matters should be answered in the best interest of the horse, with consideration for the client's position and respect to veterinary colleagues and the profession. If a person follows his or her gut feelings about the circumstances, they make the right decision in most cases. If the opportunity exists, consultation with a trusted colleague can be helpful. This person can evaluate your review of the case without personal prejudice.

TRUST IN EQUINE PRACTICE

We are in a respected position of trust with our clients. In the beginning of the veterinarian-client relationship, this trust is extended to the veterinarian because of the ethical reputation of our profession. This trust is important for us to practice effectively and efficiently. It is difficult to get things done in a proper manner if we are always looking over our shoulder and second guessing the confidence of our clients. Of course, we have all had such clients in spite of their ethical confidence. Because of the ethical reputation of our profession, the client, in most instances, extends this trust to the newly licensed veterinarian until circumstances show him or her something different.

The trust of our clients is necessary for the well-being of their horses. Veterinary medicine is significantly subjective, even though we spend a lot of energy to make it objective. When examining and treating a case, we must take the examination information and make a diagnosis, in addition to developing a treatment plan and an overall management plan for the particular disease process. It is all predicated on a judgment made at the time of the examination. The client must trust that the diagnosis is an accurate opinion and that the treatment plan is in the best interest of him or her and his or her horse and not in the veterinarian's best interest, which would not be ethical. It is important that this level of trust be maintained and principled by the veterinarian throughout the relationship with this client. Communication is the conduit for this relationship.

Trust, as defined by Stephen M.R. Covey in his book *The Speed of Trust*,[4] is the sum of character (integrity) and competence (ability). Therefore, to maintain the trust of the client, we must demonstrate consistent integrity and the ability to cope with the disease process affecting his or her horse. Integrity, ironically, can rely heavily on ability or "the lack of." As an example, if the veterinarian does not have the ability or competence to treat the horse successfully but refers the horse for the proper treatment, that veterinarian retains the trust of his client. If he or she would elect to treat the horse and be unsuccessful because of the lack of competence, he or she would lose the client's trust and likely harm the horse. In this instance, character and competence are compromised.

In this equation, character plus competence equals trust, the character component should remain constant, because we have control over our moral values and the real variable is the competence value. With good judgment and forethought, however, a veterinarian should be able to control competence too. If the expertise is lacking in a specific area, consultation or referral can be used effectively to manage the disease process. Client trust is preserved.

This, of course, is in a perfect world. It must be recognized that there can be external forces that could affect trust, such as incorrect information from the Internet or a valued friend that contradicts the veterinarian's methods. This would be a challenge of the competence factor. In this scenario, the veterinarian must rely on successful past experiences with the client (emotional bank account) and use his educational abilities to inform the client properly.

Trust that is lost because of character is more difficult to recover. If the veterinarian has the opportunity to continue with the client and can request forgiveness for the infraction, demonstrate good competence, and demonstrate renewed respect for the client, the relationship could be salvaged.

IMPLEMENTATION OF EQUINE PRACTICE ETHICS

Developing good practice ethics does not happen by chance. To have sound procedures and functions, practice leadership must led by unwavering example. This applies to a one-man practice with a small staff and to a multiple-person practice with more than one owner and many employees. All staff must understand the importance of solid ethical activities backed up by strong individual moral standards.

Leading by example, no matter how effective, must be followed up with objective discussions. Some employees do not understand the principles with just day-to-day exposure. They need to have an active thought process to understand the implications of ethics even if their moral values are credible.

ESTABLISHING CORE VALUES

One valuable exercise is for practice owners to establish a vision statement and a statement of core values for their practice. Core values are the implied or directed values or qualities that you desire to define your practice. They can be unspoken and implied through the actions of the owner. This can work if the owner has a strong personality and is communicative with the professional and lay staff. When there is more than one owner, it is important that there be direct communication among owners, first, to agree on the importance of defining their values and, second, to agree to the specifics of those values that they deem important for directing their practice. This is a congealing process that adds cohesiveness to the partnership or corporation. Once the core values are agreed on, they must be conveyed to all employees.

The process for developing core values is intense and requires honest participation by all owners, and, in some cases, it may include other stakeholders. The original collection of ideas can be gleaned from a "strengths, weaknesses, opportunities, and threats" (SWOT) exercise that includes input from the owners regarding practice.

Each owner is asked to make several entries in each of the four categories. The ideas for each category are then combined and used as a structure to develop the core values. A professional facilitator is a valuable asset for this process. He or she can ask individual questions of the owners and draw out the feelings that may not be openly expressed. It is no secret that not all equine veterinarians are forthright communicators. The facilitator can consolidate and combine thoughts to make the final document more concise. Once the core values are written and adapted by the leadership, they must be effectively communicated to all employees. They must be displayed openly where employees and owners are reminded of their content.

In addition to adding direction to the action of all employees, SWOT exercises can be used in discipline discussions and reviews with specific employees when necessary. They let everyone in the practice understand how clients and fellow employees are to be treated. They keep all stakeholders centered on their ethical and moral values.

VALUE FOR ETHICAL-BASED BUSINESSES

To get buy-in from all practice owners regarding the value of an ethical-based business may take some education. There are many examples of ethical companies that have endured the hardships of down economic cycles. There are good reference books that describe in detail the benefits of ethical business functions. Three references that would be of value in the clinic library are discussed next.

Ethics 101, by John C. Maxwell,[5] is an easy read and gives many examples of the successful operation of businesses that conduct their business based on the value of people, with the underlying theme being that all actions and conflicts can be worked out with the basic principle of the "Golden Rule."

The Speed of Trust, by Stephen M.R. Covey,[4] gives a detailed definition of and discussion about trust and how it relates to ethical behavior and credibility. It discusses gaining trust within the business and trust with the customers of the business. Discussion also surrounds the many levels of trust and the advantages associated with trust and the success of these businesses. Loss of trust is addressed also. Following is a quote from the book regarding ethics: "The increasing concern about ethics has been good for our society. Ethics (which is part of character) is foundational to trust, but by itself is insufficient. You can't have trust without ethics, but you can have ethics without trust. Trust, which encompasses ethics, is the larger idea..."[4]

Cowboy Ethics,[6] by James P. Owen with photographs by David R. Stoecklein, expounds on the loss of concern for the clients of the big Wall Street firms and offers the "Code of the West" as a starting place for the rebuilding of a more ethical culture. The pictures and the relation to the code of the developing west create a friendly read of serious nature.

The Code of the West:

1. Live each day with courage.
2. Take pride in your work.
3. Always finish what you start.
4. Do what has to be done.
5. Be tough but fair.
6. When you make a promise, keep it.
7. Ride for the brand.
8. Talk less, and say more.
9. Remember that some things are not for sale.
10. Know where to draw the line.

All three of these books would be assets for practice owner group discussions regarding ethics and how an enhanced wave of ethics could be brought into the culture of an equine practice.

SUMMARY

Ethics is a valuable standard for the structure of equine practice. It relies on sound moral character, beginning with the leaders in the practice. In simple terms, ethics can be summed up by the Golden Rule, "Whatever you want men to do to you, do also to them." The leadership in each practice regularly needs to review its role in promoting ethical standards. This is not new information but deserves to be revisited with emphasis at this particular time in our society. Many big businesses and their leaders, in addition to our highest levels of political leaders, are not performing up to the standards we hold dear in our profession. Nothing less than commitment to grass root stability offers any hope to reverse those actions.

REFERENCES

1. The History of the AAEP. The second 25 years 1980–2004. American Association of Equine Practitioners; Lexington, Kentucky. p. 27.
2. Webster's New World Dictionary College Edition, 1958. World Publishing Company.
3. American Association of Equine Practitioners 2009 resource guide and membership directory. p. 23–33.
4. Covey SMR. The speed of trust. New York (NY): Free Press; 2006. p. 30.
5. Maxwell JC. Ethics 101. New York: Time Warner Book Group.
6. Owen JP, Stoecklein DR. Cowboy ethics. Stoecklein Publishing. p. 24.

Marketing Your Equine Practice

Robert P. Magnus, DVM, MBA

KEYWORDS

- Equine marketing • Equine business management

As licensed working veterinarians, we have completed 4 years of undergraduate work, 4 additional years of veterinary medical school, possibly an internship, and then perhaps a residency program. During all these years of formal education, there are few, if any, opportunities or courses to help us develop the business skills necessary for financial success. We remain so focused on the clinical practice of veterinary medicine that strategy and planning often fall by the wayside, putting the future of our practices at risk. In fact, in our profession, the concept of marketing is often deemed potentially unethical. Striking a balance between providing excellent health care and marketing is a challenge, but it can be done.

Marketing a veterinary practice is so much more than merely making decisions regarding telephone book and newspaper advertisements, which sponsorship banners to hang at the show grounds, or the creation of promotional packages to offer to clients. Although these are legitimate marketing tactics and they do play a role in the overall practice marketing strategy and plan, we must begin to see marketing from a different more interactive perspective. When we are effectively marketing ourselves, we are participating in the ongoing process of determining and anticipating customer needs, creating ways to satisfy those customer needs, and targeting the appropriate market in alignment with our strategy and skills. Marketing allows us the opportunity to investigate and develop new ideas to satisfy the horse owner while we continue to deliver necessary patient care; this is "marketing in action." By reaching the right market niche with the proper product, we are allowed the opportunity to enhance our profession by providing necessary care and education.

We are often faced with questions regarding marketing our equine practices, and it is likely that we are so busy with the day-to-day work of our profession that we have little time to investigate possible answers and options. For example, where do you find resources to help in promoting your equine business? How much of the expense of marketing is likely to be offset by improved profitability? How does marketing tie into an exit strategy? What are the demographics of my area's horse population? What is my future workforce likely to look like? Is my practice positioned to adapt to future changes? Can I afford to retire according to my own time frame, and when and how do I want to exit this wonderful profession?

Wisconsin Equine Clinic and Hospital, 39151 Delafield Road, Oconomowoc, WI 53066, USA
E-mail address: ultraeq@aol.com

Vet Clin Equine 25 (2009) 463–473
doi:10.1016/j.cveq.2009.07.008
0749-0739/09/$ – see front matter

These questions may seem daunting. Attaining your personal and professional goals is possible, however, and good planning and marketing should be at the heart of the overall business planning process. Ultimately, this requires you to take the time to plan strategically for the future. The most common responses to this statement are "I don't have the time" and "I don't have the kind of resources that are available to larger practices." My response is that you must make the time to deal with these issues and you cannot afford not to deal with them. There are simple inexpensive approaches to marketing your practice. Planning your future and effectively integrating marketing strategies into your practice can help you to reach your business potential and increase your practice profitability.

Developing and implementing a marketing strategy requires, first, the creation of a roadmap to enhance the value of your product in the eyes of your customers and, second, capture of a portion of that effort (profits) through pricing. Traditional marketing strategies use analysis models to help create and capture value, in addition to using processes to sustain that value in your business. To begin this process, you must analyze multiple factors that are in and out of your control. This framework involves five primary activities: (1) selecting the target market, (2) providing the right services to the right customer, (3) developing a strategic plan, (4) using tactics and tools to achieve your correct position in the marketplace, and (5) continued active monitoring and adjustments to the plan. Throughout this article, these five activities are addressed as part of an overall marketing strategy process. The key to this whole process lies in understanding your customers' needs and their buying behavior.

In some respects, marketing uses an entirely different language in and of itself. **Box 1** lists some of the terms and definitions commonly used in the marketing industry, which can serve as a reference. In this article, the author provides an overview of marketing analysis using the "three C's" and "four P's" framework examples. The author also introduces the concept of customer relationship management (CRM). Finally, he lays out 10 practical steps to help you start the process of developing a strategic marketing process or framework to market your equine practice effectively.

"THREE C'S" ANALYSIS

Customers, company, and competition are three entities that can be used as business indicators. It is important to measure the individual and group attributes of your customers, your own company, and your competition. This analysis framework examines internal and external factors and their effects on your equine veterinary practice.

To help you to define your target market and desired positioning before major decisions are made, ask yourself the following questions:

Customers
- Who are my customers?
- Why do they use my services?
- What are the demographics of horse owners and horses in my market area?
- Are there service and product needs that are not being met?
- Are there opportunities for growth and expansion?
- Who are my good/profitable accounts?

Company
- What are the strengths and weaknesses?
- What are the core competencies of this business today?
- What are the short-and long-term goals and vision for the business?
- What opportunities exist in our unique practice area?

Box 1
Marketing and communication terms

Awareness: the percentage of the population or target market that is aware of the existence of a given brand or company defines the market awareness.

Brand: a mixture of attributes, tangible and intangible, symbolized in a trademark, which, if managed properly, creates value and influence. A brand is composed of five elements: position, promise, personality, story, and associations. Most important is a brand that is portrayed consistently.

Core competencies: relates to a company's particular area of skill and competence that best contributes to its ability to compete.

Demographics: the description of outward traits that characterize a group of people, such as age, gender, nationality, marital status, education, occupation, or income. Decisions on market segmentation are often based on demographic data.

Differentiation: creation or demonstration of unique characteristics in a company's products or brands compared with those of its competitors.

Focus group: a qualitative research technique in which a group of approximately eight people is invited to a neutral venue to discuss a given subject. The principle is the same as an in-depth interview, except that group dynamics help to make the discussion livelier and more wide-ranging. Qualitative groups enable the researcher to probe deeper into specific areas of interest (eg, the nature of commitment to a brand). The result adds richer texture to the understanding of broader data (eg, quantitative), which may point out general trends or observation. This technique is also known as group discussion.

Goal: a concrete short-term point of measurement that the business unit intends to meet in pursuit of its objectives. An overall objective converts into specific short-run goals.

Marketing: a social and managerial function that attempts to create, expand, and maintain a collection of customers. In a nutshell, marketing is any activity that aims to make humans behave in a desired manner. Marketing, as suggested by the American Marketing Association, is the process of planning and executing the conception, pricing, promotion, and distribution of ideas, goods, and services to create exchanges that satisfy individual and organizational objectives.

Marketing communications: describe the methods marketing uses to communicate to the target audiences what is identified as important to the sales process. When prices are all approximately the same, customers buy what they have always bought—the brand that is most familiar and comfortable. Marketing communications strive to make brands familiar and comfortable.

Market segment: a group of customers who (1) share the same needs and values, (2) can be expected to respond in much the same way to a company's offering, and (3) command enough purchasing power to be of strategic importance to the company.

Market share: a company's share of total sales of a given category of product in a given market. This can be expressed in terms of volume (how many units sold) or value (the worth of units sold).

Mission: the purpose for which the organization exists, or the answer to the question, "What business are we in?" The corporate mission statement, with a broad focus and a customer orientation, provides management with a sense of purpose.

Niche marketing: marketing adapted to the needs, wishes, and expectations of small precisely defined groups of individuals. A form of market segmentation but aimed at small segments. Niche marketing characteristically uses selective media.

Objective: marketing and communication objectives are simply "what needs to be accomplished." Objectives should be SMART (specific, measurable, achievable, realistic, and time-tabled).

Strategy: how are we going to accomplish the objective? This is typically the key to any plan and should always be developed before tactics.

Tactic: specific actions used to implement a strategy.

Target audience or market: a specific market segment that should be targeted for marketing and communication efforts (eg, horse owners who show in the Ocala area).

Vision: a short, succinct, and inspiring statement of what the organization intends to become and to achieve at some point in the future, which is often stated in competitive terms. This is the expression of the ultimate aim to which the business aspires.

Competition

- Who are the competitors in the area?
- What are the competitors' strengths and weakness?
- What services do I offer that I have in common and that are different?
- What is the competitors' reputation?

Dig deep and explore these questions and other attributes in the "three C's" analysis. **Fig. 1** provides a conceptual view of this analysis framework. Pay close attention to the last two elements in the diagram: evaluation of options and decisions and implementation. These are the essential steps that should be taken after completion of your market and customer analyses that define the success or failure of a marketing strategy.

"FOUR P'S" ANALYSIS

In the analysis of pricing, place, promotion, and product, pricing philosophy drives the revenue side of the equation and the place, promotion, and product are subtracted from the cost structure, resulting in a profit or loss for your business. Your pricing strategy and the value provided by the services or products that you sell are the foundation of marketing your practice.

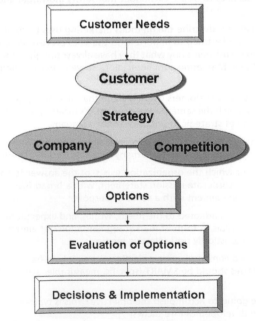

Fig. 1. "Three C's" analysis framework.

Price is a sensitive subject in the equine veterinary industry. It is the most important component available to improving your company's profitability. To a large extent, the target customer's perception of the value of your services represents the maximum price the customer is willing to pay. Veterinary medicine, in general, is considered to be price-inelastic. Price changes do not have a large effect on consumer purchases. In essence, veterinary services and products are not as price-sensitive as is the case when someone is shopping for a television set or another commodity product. The customer buys because of the value of the service you offer (treatment for their horse), in large part, based on the trust and relationship between the veterinarian, client, and patient.

Place (channels) are the delivery components to selling your services and products. What avenues are best for your practice? Should you focus your business on field service or ambulatory care, or are you positioned in the marketplace to be a referral hospital? In these two examples, there is a significant cost (overhead) disparity and profitability margin differential to consider. Advances in technology and the Internet have also created new marketing opportunities, such as delivery of pharmaceutics directly to your clients.

Promotion of your products and services can follow different paths. You must communicate with customers to foster their awareness of the services and products that your practice offers. For example, if you offer elective surgery and your farm accounts do not know that you have this capability, clients are going to seek out your competitors to fill that need. Do your clients know what services you offer? Do they know your areas of expertise? Once you have these answers, decide how much and what types of promotional activities are needed to target the appropriate customer segment.

Products (service) offered should ideally be established by the customers' needs and characterized by the desired attributes of the services or products sold. These tastes and preferences have a cost basis. Are you meeting your customers' needs, and does your company have the resources (eg, technology, labor, expertise) to capture that aspect of the market? Value can be delivered by several vehicles, such as the service itself, the brand name, the company reputation, the veterinarian's reputation, service care, emergency care accessibility, therapeutic results, and word-of-mouth references.

CUSTOMER RELATIONSHIP MANAGEMENT

CRM requires developing a better understanding of your current and potential customers and, based on this information, maximizing all opportunities to influence their buying behavior. The goal of CRM is to realize the full profit potential of your practice. Simply put, there are three general approaches to CRM:

1. Find more: Has your practice targeted all the potential customers in your marketplace?
2. Win more: Are you maximizing the full purchasing potential of existing customers?
3. Keep more: Are you retaining your best customers? Have you developed deep customer loyalty, or are you just the best of the available options in your practice area?

Understanding the key drivers of your customers' buying behavior is essential. Horse owners' existing needs drive their motivation to seek your services. For CRM to be effective, you must:

- Identify your customer's relevant motivations and needs.
- Assess the importance of these motivations and needs.
- Identify your customer's choice process (buying behavior).

CRM is also about managing customer relationships and building loyalty. It is an ongoing management process designed to understand your customers' buying behavior. Using current advances in technology can help to streamline this process and allow you to analyze easily the effectiveness and profitability of different marketing strategies.

Creating a customer database using current veterinary software or other CRM software can help you to focus your marketing effort toward different segments of your customer base. For example, it would be costly and ineffective to send a mailing to all your clients regarding a reproductive seminar if 80% of your customers are sport horse accounts. Having a detailed and comprehensive database allows you to segment your clients based on multiple attributes. Listed next are a few customer segmentation ideas to consider:

- Discipline: performance horse, pleasure horse, race horse, other
- Breed: Arabian, quarter horse, hunter/jumper, other
- Services used: breeding, preventive health care, sport horse, surgery, dentistry, other
- Top 50 customers by annual revenue: current year, comparative annual analysis
- Top 15 referral veterinarians: number of cases, revenue generation, other

How you manage your customer relationships translates into different levels of customer satisfaction and loyalty. You can choose how you want to interact with your customers. The entire process starts with the establishment of a detailed and comprehensive database and using that information to attract new customers, convert them, and retain them.

Fig. 2 illustrates the general CRM framework and analysis process starting with creating the database. Working on each of these areas improves customer loyalty and gives you a better understanding of your target market.

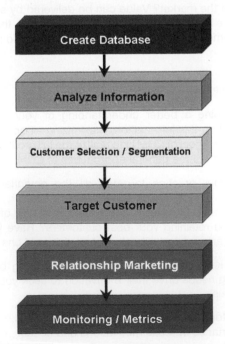

Fig. 2. CRM framework.

According to the *Merriam Webster's Dictionary*, marketing is the process or technique of promoting, selling, and distributing a product or service. **Fig. 3** illustrates an overall marketing framework to guide you in the process. Begin by assessing your goals, and then focus on analyzing your customers and target market. Next, formulate a comprehensive marketing plan. Finally, monitor and adjust your marketing activities based on changes and new opportunities in the practice area.

Business models, frameworks, and analytic tools are useful methods to help you develop a strategic marketing plan. In the next section, the author takes a practical approach to planning using "10 steps of marketing your equine practice," which is a great place to start.

Professional Goals and Practice Goals

As practitioners, we strive to provide quality medicine and great service while obtaining the best possible results for our clients. Equally important is the need to evaluate your current business status and better define future personal and professional goals. Many practitioners know this, but putting it into play is challenging. Make goal setting a priority. Set aside time so that you can achieve this outcome. Whether you are a solo practitioner or in a group practice, ask the following questions:

- What are the core values of this practice?
- What are we good at, individually and as a group?
- What does each of us enjoy doing in our veterinary profession?
- Where do we envision this practice to be in 3, 5, and 10 years?
- How, when, and under what terms do I want to retire?
- Am I happy professionally? If not, what do I need to do to be satisfied in this practice?

Answer and discuss these questions. This is the first step in planning for the future and developing a sound marketing strategy to help you achieve your personal and professional goals. Without a defined vision, it is difficult and often frustrating when you must decide which marketing tools to use and where to spend limited resources.

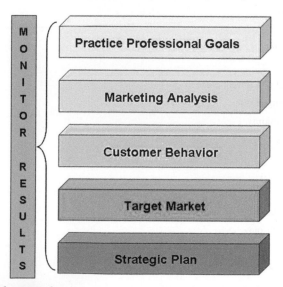

Fig. 3. Marketing framework.

> **Box 2**
> **Marketing tools and tactics**
>
> The list of possible tactics is almost limitless, especially as new technology is introduced. Clients have access to a lot of information, but the key is to ensure that any touch point they have supports your message and brand. Consistency is key. You can use tactics from this list or develop your own for use in your marketing communications plans.
>
> National advertising
>
> Special events
>
> Billboards
>
> Regional advertising
>
> Trade show booth
>
> Focus groups
>
> Local advertising
>
> Open house
>
> Surveys
>
> Classified advertising
>
> Media events
>
> Word-of-mouth marketing
>
> Radio advertising
>
> Continuing education seminars
>
> Testimonials
>
> Special advertising
>
> Partnerships
>
> Feature stories
>
> Basic direct mail postcard
>
> Sponsorships
>
> Special promotions
>
> Direct mail series
>
> Training videotape/digital versatile disc
>
> Wellness programs
>
> Three-dimensional direct mail piece
>
> Informational compact disc
>
> Logo clothing/premium
>
> Statement stuffers
>
> Web site updates
>
> Items (eg, caps, shirts)
>
> Special invitations
>
> Web banners and advertising
>
> Point-of-purchase display
>
> Press release
>
> Clinic information packets
>
> Giveaways

Editorial

Brochure

Magnets, pens, notepads

Advertorial

Sell sheets

Bumper stickers

First-to-know informational letter

Flyers

Business cards

Newsletters

Product detailers

Posters

Thank-you cards

Magazine articles

Social media

Internal "Self-Evaluation"

What are the characteristics of your current practice environment? Is it friendly, helpful, and efficient or confrontational with poor customer service? A comprehensive internal evaluation of all positions and job responsibilities is critical to your success. Identifying staffing issues, support staff expertise, and your ability to expand plays an important role in implementing marketing ideas. Great marketing campaigns are only great if you have the resources and commitment of your team to put them into place and make them work.

Area Demographics

An accurate assessment of your practice area demographics is imperative. A strong knowledge of your current horse population coupled with the ability to project the future direction of your client base (database analysis) can help you in this process. Your goals and aspirations may not be attainable if the economic environment is changing and not aligned with your goals. Can your clients afford the level of service (price)? What is the average household income in the counties where you provide care? Are you focusing your marketing efforts in the proper region of your practice? Sound information is the key to success here.

Target Market: Perception Versus Reality

Most of us believe that we provide a great value and service to our horse clients. We work long hours, are passionate about our careers, and achieve great results. Do our clients feel the same about us as we think they do? Who is your target market? Current evidence suggests horse owners are not as loyal as we would like to think. Do your clients know what services and expertise you and your practice offer? A recent trend in veterinary medicine shows that clients have started to "boutique" their veterinary service needs. Your practice may be missing an opportunity to increase its revenue because clients are seeking the services of other professionals, simply because they are not aware of your abilities or the services offered through your practice. Unfortunately, this seemingly innocuous lack of communication has a substantial impact on the client's perception of you and what your practice has to offer. To be effective, you must inform current and potential clients about new services (profit centers) you have created, and more than once. Set yourself apart from your competitors with the services you offer, and make sure you let everyone know.

Understanding Customer Buying Behavior

This is one of the most important and difficult aspects in the analysis process. Why do horse owners use you instead of the practice down the road? What are the important attributes that drive the customer to buy your services? Is it your friendly service, emergency response time, special skills, medical results, pricing, or other factors that differentiate you and your practice from the competition?

Strategic Plan

Without a solid marketing plan for short-term (first 12 months) and long-term (3–5 years) growth of your business, it is easy to waste time, money, and staff resources. The planning process begins with ownership and then must incorporate your support staff. A shared vision of the practice is necessary for success. Time spent developing this process is crucial and drives the entire marketing process.

Tactics and Tools

What tools work best? There is no easy answer to this question. Marketing tools are planned pieces or activities that target your goals in promoting the practice. What works in Palm Beach, Florida, may not be effective in Lincoln, Nebraska. Understanding your "current" and potential "new" client base is paramount in selecting those tools that can achieve a positive outcome. Some common and effective tools include newsletters, wellness programs, open houses, statement stuffers, brochures, fliers or "sell sheets," educational seminars, press releases, and proactive Web pages. The lists of possible tools are infinite; select those items that best promote your business and elicit a positive response from your clientele. One way to do this is to survey a target group of customers. **Box 2** presents a list of tools and tactics to consider.

Costs…Budget

It is easy to spend money on flashy advertisements or campaigns to promote your business. It is more difficult but rewarding to stick to your strategic plan. If you have been thoughtful and careful in creating your individual plan, you have incorporated realistic expectations and benefiting from cost-efficient marketing expenses. Design a simple 18-month marketing spreadsheet on an Excel document. Define the costs, number of pieces, target market, and timing of your strategic action plan. How much time is needed for planning, implementation, and monitoring of every marketing effort? Can you afford to spend the resources needed to implement your marketing plan, or should your plan and expectations be modified?

Action Plan

You have developed the plan within your budget and focused on your goals. Before moving forward, consider other factors as well. For example, is the timing right for your market area to act on your plan? Are you sending a consistent real message throughout all your marketing pieces? Are your support staff and veterinary staff on board and fully informed? Can your support staff handle the additional responsibilities presented with the new marketing initiative? When you can comfortably answer "yes" to these questions, go for it.

Monitoring

You have just spent a tremendous amount of time and money and launched a marketing program. Is it working? When are you likely to see the results of all the time and money spent? What tools work best? Monitoring your results is one of the most challenging aspects of marketing. Most practices begin to see a positive response as early as 12 months after initiation of the program, but it may take as long as 18 to 24 months before you realize a return on your investment. Make sure to define objective parameters that measure the response to the goals you developed in the planning process. Also, recognize that several aspects of marketing are difficult and sometimes impossible to measure. Decision making is difficult without a measurable metric in place to assess the outcome of your original marketing decision.

SUMMARY

The take-home message in marketing your equine practice is simple: understand your position in the target market and the buying behavior of your current and prospective customers. Time well spent on analysis and evaluation of options can maximize customer value in the services and products you offer. This allows you to capture profit and to attain your personal and professional goals as an equine practitioner.

Design of a Multifaceted Referral Equine Hospital

Peter C. Bousum, VMD

KEYWORDS

* Multifaceted Practices * Management of Practices

Most veterinarians, sometime during their career, entertain thoughts of belonging to or owning a multifaceted referral hospital and practice. In recent years, many of our educational institutions have recognized the need for business education. However, business education is not the primary objective of a veterinary school and is typically not the forefront of interest of students already taxed with massive information overload. While we may subconsciously feel a need for a lifestyle less burdened by the pressures of work, our real passion during the formative years is the science of our profession. Recent graduates may typically choose to either take a position as an associate or pursue further specialty training. In spite of caveats and veiled signals from those established in practice, we tend to put business matters on the back burner. We think we can always develop business acumen later in life. After all, the handling of business matters must be simple compared to dealing with the intense competition and highly complex education we have just completed. We assume that organizational and leadership skills are easy, that business relationships are simple to maintain, and that, if we just position ourselves in the workplace, the money will come in easily and the minor details will work themselves out.

Most of us develop our nonveterinary skills only after finding ourselves the unpleasant choice of taking on an unwanted responsibility or facing failure. The authors of the articles in this issue have either felt the fire of such situations or have chosen to selectively fill the need for advice and leadership. Key words and paradigms mentioned include *leadership*, *strategic planning*, *communication*, *branding*, *internal* and *external mission statements*, *shifting paradigms*, *accountability*, *tax and succession planning*, *partnership and employment agreements*, and *compensation*. Many others are mentioned as well, producing in most of us a reflex of involuntary sleep and avoidance. Incredibly, and understandably, these don't become meaningful until they actually provide significant results. If you are considering a state-of-the-art multifaceted practice, nothing could be more important than to devote your time to understanding and applying these terms and concepts.

Medical professionals (veterinarians, physicians, dentists) who decide to form a business assume a somewhat unique dynamic: They are immediately and

The MidAtlantic Equine Medical Center, PO Box 188, 40 Frontage Road, Ringoes, NJ 08551, USA
E-mail address: pbousum@starband.net

Vet Clin Equine 25 (2009) 475–488
doi:10.1016/j.cveq.2009.08.002
0749-0739/09/$ – see front matter © 2009 Elsevier Inc. All rights reserved.

unequivocally separated by their position in society; they must complete long and rigorous training to acquire an accredited degree; they must pass the scrutiny of various state and professional boards; they must be duly licensed; and they are thus elevated to the position of doctor. This separates them from their employees in the business and from many people in society. No one can start out as the classic "delivery boy" and move to the top (as with the corporate legends) unless they undergo the same education and certification as a doctor. Thus, without a structure that allows less skilled people to move up the corporate ladder, discipline at a veterinarian practice is often difficult to maintain. The doctor, like the lawyer, almost always considers himself on the same level professionally as his immediate peers and assumes an equal right to make decisions regardless of ownership. Employees, meanwhile, tend to see no differences among the roles of the individual doctors. This is an important fact and will be discussed later.

Fig. 1 shows one example of a basic map for the structure of a "multifaceted equine hospital." Each of these topics and subtopics encompass volumes of information, the subject of many books and deliberations far too complex for this article. However, managing a large practice is more than a full-time job for one veterinarian or partner. The management needs are exponentially greater in a large hospital practice than in smaller entities. Some veterinarians placed in leadership positions have recognized the need for formal education and have obtained a master of business administration degree when faced with the role of managing partner. This article provides some thoughts about key issues involved in maintaining a large practice. The process is dynamic and more information is available every day. The formation of "study groups" and recent recognition by the American Association of Equine Practitioners, universities, and publications provide avenues of awareness that have raised the level of business proficiency and success among veterinary practices. Equine veterinarians need the continued involvement of these organizations and others in issues related to business practices.

DECIDING TO BUILD: INITIALLY AN IDEA?

Most decisions to commit to a large multifaceted facility are stimulated by several factors: economic opportunity, rapid growth of a multidoctor practice, inherent need in the community, and, most importantly, a desire to practice at a different level. The process begins as an idea and then leads to a task that may evolve over many years. Jim Collins, a highly successful disciplinarian and corporate guru who had written several bestselling books on corporate issues, was entertaining the thought of forming a larger multifaceted consulting business when he heeded the words of one of his mentors, the late Peter Drucker, a pioneer in social and management strategies: "If you want to build ideas first and foremost then you must not build a big organization because you will wind up managing that organization."[1] Taking on the task of building a large multifaceted practice and facility will change your lifestyle precipitously. Your role as a practitioner will diminish and your time for other outside endeavors will plummet markedly for many years until the entity evolves into a solid organization. While early contemplation and research is necessary, the venture ultimately requires a strong, highly motivated commitment.

Economic Opportunity

Most who consider the prospect of building a large multifaceted practice are convinced that, by supplying the horse community with additional services (local emergency care, such as that for colic surgery and medical emergencies, and intensive care) or high-end diagnostic capabilities (magnetic resonance, CT, scintigraphy,

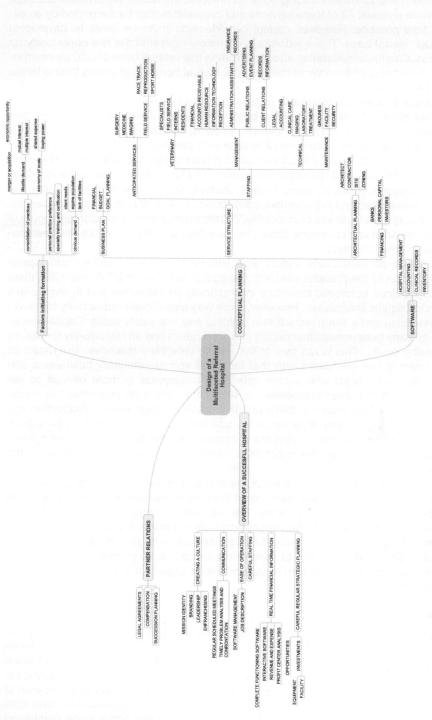

Fig. 1. Basic map for the structure of a "multifaceted equine hospital."

and others) and innovative cutting-edge techniques, the facility will produce substantially more revenue. All of these services and capabilities may be supported by an existing field practice. However, careful consideration must be given to developing a robust referral base. These individuals ultimately represent the real opportunity for success. Careful consideration about cultivating this referral base should be incorporated in the basic philosophy of the practice. Mutual benefit and strong trust is tantamount to success.

Financial modeling is absolutely necessary. Most veterinarians embarking in business will already have established a basic knowledge of income statements, cash flow analysis, and forecasting. However, in terms of business complexity, there is an exponential difference between a smaller field practice and a major hospital. Any consideration must begin with an analysis that is as detailed as possible. A few additional considerations will be expenses involving initial capital investment and added costs (mortgage, taxes, equipment loans, staffing, insurance, and maintenance). For both the uninitiated and experienced, a seasoned consultant is an absolute necessity. A well thought out business plan requires enfranchising much of the staff and hours of regular meetings and communication. The basic business plan structure has been discussed in other chapters.

Economic considerations should also include the cost of money and careful consideration of the financial trends in the equine industry. In 2008 and 2009, there was an obvious economic downturn in practically all industries and in most areas related to equine businesses. However, there was also a great opportunity for favorable financing and a sharp reduction in building and real estate costs. Capital investment in many businesses often results in a solid return and an opportunity for rapidly increasing equity. This is not true of the equine veterinary business. The return on investment is low compared with that for small animal veterinary businesses and real estate associated with equine veterinary businesses is more difficult to sell than that of many other businesses. A substantial return on investment to stockholders may not be available until a practice reaches a high level of production and efficiency. This of course depends on the size and extent of the facility. Where large amounts of unencumbered capital are available, the cash flow requirements may be greatly diminished and offer substantial salary and bonus considerations to the shareholders.

Future trends in the equine veterinary field may see the formation of mergers and acquisitions. This has already been noted in small animal veterinary businesses and has been successful in many cases. The rationale is similar: the potential to offer more and better services, the benefits of economies of scale, and opportunities to split the cost of large-ticket items and reduce redundancy. A larger merged company also can offer a more efficient way to transfer capital and value (smoother exit strategy), a constantly troubling issue with equine practices (Owen McCafferty, CPA, personal communication, 2007).

Demographic Need

Dr Bob Magnus in his article discusses marketing and the importance of studying and maintaining the catchment. This is an excellent discussion that offers advice on developing sound criteria for establishing a facility. In the past, many if not most facilities were built with little serious consideration for factors associated with the demographic needs. They were often built out of a desire to practice in such a facility or because of discontent with a current position. Once established most veterinarians have little desire to leave their immediate practice area. Rarely, a practice may be purchased by a remotely located doctor with the immediate intention of expanding the practice into a facility. Present economic situations suggest that knee-jerk development may not be prudent. The equine population is growing more slowly now than in the last 2 decades. The veterinary production pie has become markedly smaller. Unless we can offer better, more efficient, or distinctively innovative services, we face the possibility of stagnation. As stressed in other articles, perceived value is largely relative to economic times. Discretional spending has significantly diminished and is likely to remain tight for some time. Clients appear to be spending mostly when there is a substantial need and not on preventative medicine. During these tight-spending conditions, critical care will not likely be influenced as much as elective procedures.

Personal Agenda

Many equine practitioners are highly trained in specialized fields. These individuals have developed an expertise that may often be best used in a larger facility or referral practice. Understandably, these people have a burning desire to use their expertise and grow intellectually, often on the cutting edge of the industry. Those who desire a position in a large facility would like to have a broad support staff and structure to follow many of their cases from start to finish. Others see an advantage of the readily available staff and structure for implementing efficiencies related to, for example, billing, accounting, computer services, maintenance, on-call relief, and office space. Still others see the advantage of a group practice with broad intellectual support and experience and the ready availability of high-ticket in-house diagnostics and laboratory.

A desire for a more flexible lifestyle is a strong reason to join or form a large practice. Family emergencies, vacations, and other extended leaves are much easier to facilitate in large practices, where many practitioners are available to temporarily handle the work of an absent practitioner. Also, insurance, continuing education, and retirement plans are routinely offered in a larger practice. As the practice grows, it becomes economically feasible to employ more staff for after-hour needs, which results in more free time for the principals and other staff.

Most importantly, a larger facility or practice enables most doctors to focus on their primary work as veterinarians and not be burdened by the constant needs of managing a smaller entity. The exception is the doctor or doctors who accept the responsibility of management whether on a full-time or part-time basis. Efficiency allows for more individual production with fewer hours, often giving the practitioner a substantially better lifestyle than those who must remain on call at all times.

Partnerships

The topic of partners could produce several books alone. The decision to expand to a large practice with a facility often must be made with a partner and may in many cases depend on the formation of a partnership or on expanding a partnership. The choice of partners is an extremely important decision. It is often said that a partnership is more difficult than a marriage. Before the hospital is created, the primary individuals involved must be carefully chosen and a partnership formed. Partners are often extremely competent and understanding individuals with a great deal of experience in veterinary medicine and deep personal relationships. Even so, completely functional partnerships are almost unheard of. This is not to discourage the decision to expand, only to suggest that a solid relationship takes a great deal of effort, similar to that required in a marriage. Professional help should also be considered before signing on the dotted line, including personality testing and counseling. Bumps in the road are likely and should be anticipated. Compensation, production, and leadership responsibilities will always be part of dynamic policy changes and only individuals with the ability to reason with each other should be considered. A culture of strong interpersonal communication is necessary and will be discussed later.

INFORMATION AND DECISION-MAKING

Management of a large practice requires careful attention to structure and constant monitoring of information and trends. A strong understanding of business accounting and management is essential. Equally important is real-time access to information through well-designed computer systems and regular staff communication. Financial decision-making must be supported with historical and predicted analysis and focal modeling. Good information is necessary for practically every decision in the business, including decisions involving expanding, staffing, purchasing, working with clients and cases, determining compensation, choosing benefits, and, often, veterinary care itself. With a smaller entity, such decisions can often be postponed until the end of the month, until support staff has time to compile the necessary information, until the computer or accounting system can be accessed, or until the accountant or attorney supplies the necessary papers and reports. In a large practice, these delays cause serious issues and can severely reduce efficiency. Delays in making decisions result not only in inefficiency, but can also lead to immediate and long-term discontent among the staff and may even result in legal entanglements.

Understanding Business

I would highly recommend that all principals in a larger practice (partners and managers) pursue a course in business management similar to those offered before entering into the multifaceted venture.[2] A good understanding of income statements and balance sheets is a necessity. They should also be versed in budgeting and corporate structure. Legal agreements, such as partnership agreements, leases, buy-sell agreements, and documents related to limited liability companies, C corporations, and S corporations, all can have a role in the way a business is structured and operated. Regular review of the understanding is necessary, but often ignored or placed on the back burner because of other responsibilities.

The process and dynamics of partnerships will most likely change as the profession matures. There will always be a better way. However, decisions and commitments must be made in a timely fashion if the entity is to survive and grow.

Systematic Information Production, Data Gathering, and Output

A discussion of medical records has been presented in another article. However, this information should be integrated with a strong financial program as well. A large hospital today should make terminals available throughout the hospital and field service and have software that enables paperless operations. Most systems have traditionally been able to offer information regarding an animal on a chronologic and not episodic basis, similar to information on a paper hospital record. Some of the systems now offer, in addition to that capability, the white board (treatment scheduler), which segregates the information into a real-time hospital record and has the same form as a paper folder. Treatments can be scheduled and marked off at the time and place of treatment or procedure. Billing and inventory reduction can be produced with one keystroke, producing a real-time compilation of charges and expenses with a cost-of-goods system. Billing profiles, reports, and documentation with treatment scheduling can be generated at admission or scheduling and modified throughout the episode. Discharge instructions and client communication can be produced from any terminal in a few seconds, creating a timely response and constantly updating costs. These capabilities make for much higher efficiencies, compared to the traditional method of hospital operations, and enable tasks to be done with fewer staff so that more veterinary time can be devoted to production. The typical case should be completely finished at the time of discharge and not weeks later when the time is available. Such changes are universally met with staff resistance, which is why implementation often fails even in those practices that have the installed capability. This resistance costs a typical practice a great deal of production and profit.

Profit Center Accounting and Information

Few of the systems available integrate the veterinary module with the accounting system. Any hospital should either purchase an existing system with this capability or one that is near completion. Profit centers are often wrongly mistaken as revenue centers. A revenue center only shows the dollars generated and is not synonymous with profit. Many expensive procedures with a high overhead may produce revenue but result in little or no profit. Others may have little overhead and large profit (lameness examinations, prepurchased services). The ideal computer system should provide the capabilities to divide the hospital into profit centers by reporting the income and expense involved for these specific entities or departments. Smaller models can be used for specific components of a profit center (digital radiographs or MRI analysis in the imaging department). This reporting should be provided in real time if possible to assist the manager in making serious decisions in a timely manner regarding, for example, personnel, investments, upgrades, and facility needs. This data can be reported as individual (departmental) income statements and can be easily graphed and compared with data from other departments or profit centers (**Fig. 2**). In **Fig. 2**, the summary trends of profit in the sample hospital showed rather smooth trends for all the income statement totals and irregular trends in individual departments. By tracing the individual trends to their separate income statements (profit and loss), a manager can easily discover the reason for such trends and make corrections or adjustments to produce more profits. This information is not available in systems that don't easily integrate the veterinary and accounting software.[3]

This system also depends on a dynamic cost-of-goods system where inventory must be taken out of the system at the point of treatment or use. This can be done for treatment procedures and for consumable noninventory goods, such as toilet paper and towels. Because this method shows the actual loss of individual items in a timely fashion and the subsequent revenue reduction, this is the only way to effectively control inventory and justify regular manual inventories. Most individuals only count their inventory against the purchases, which is good only for adjusting the balance sheet and net worth. It does not show the real loss nor suggest where the loss has occurred. This system also depends on careful addition of inventory through timely recognition of purchase orders and statements.

Our hospital's system has included a cost-of-goods component for at least 3 years and a departmental accounting component for 6 years. Providing these capabilities takes a great deal of initial setup and ongoing diligence, but it can be done. We feel that it is the only way to properly manage a hospital and the decisions based on information provided by these additional capabilities have resulted in significantly greater profit. A word about veterinary software systems: We often choose systems because of one or two items that catch our eye and impress us. These can be anything from a great appointment scheduler, to impressive graphics, to integrated accounting. The average user employs about 20% of the system's capabilities and takes little time to study the modules. Every system requires a great deal of time and work to maximize its capabilities. A larger hospital needs a full-time information technology

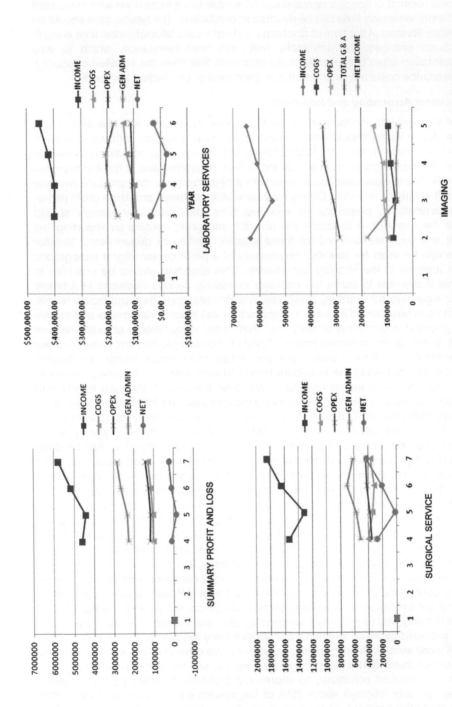

Fig. 2. Several Profit and Loss graphs showing the summary (overall) and individual profit center trends. Note that profit centers include revenue and expense data and that they do not necessarily follow the summary trends. This is a very helpful way to monitor expenses and make informed decisions in the financial management and investment. Each variance in the profit center lines can easily be explained by referring to the detailed individual P & L data.

person with a number of additional highly trained individuals to constantly mentor and update the remaining staff. It is worth the effort to spend a great deal of time exploring these systems and working with them for a number of days before making a decision on change.

Even though we were not trained to be retailers, it is more the norm than the exception that retail goods serve as a profit center in many practices. Thus, retailing deserves some consideration. While we should be expected to charge for our services and expertise similar to physicians, the profession has long held retailing as part of the formula for business success. In many practices, retailing represents a significant part of the gross revenue and is assumed to be profitable. However, a serious analysis of the business aspects of carrying inventory versus sales and cash flow consistently shows that there is very little profit in a high-risk business that requires constant attention and staffing. Many factors put pressure on profits. These include costs related to maintaining inventory and bad debts; cost changes; and competition from Internet and local stores.. There are currently designs for focal Internet credit card sales that will minimize much of the risk. However, moves to do more retailing business via the Internet places us in direct competition with each other and has little to do with our core services. As trends continue, we may be faced with even more downward price pressure and find retailing no longer profitable. The profession must find an answer to this possibility or we will find ourselves mired in a situation that will be difficult to exit. We could lose access to modern methods of name recognition.

We are often compelled to lower our prices to some of our best clients because our competitor offers it at a substantially lower price. This is rarely because they are better business people or because they are buying it cheaper. They are simply reacting to market pressure whether real or imagined. Kelly Lyons, in his book *The One Percent Solution*, clearly shows methodology for price changes and has relatively seamless models for predicting change to return on investment relative to sales. It is an easy way to see just how much influence price and total sales have on the bottom line with expenses changing slightly or staying the same. We often use this model in our staff meetings when we contemplate price changes and marketing of many items.[4]

Modeling

A common decision that we must make is the decision to purchase new equipment or add personnel. Many models for these decisions are readily available and can be purchased from one of the more prominent consultants in our field. My personal choice is a free download from Excel for Business.[5] This model can be used for many decisions and can be tweaked as needed. Similar information can be made from your personal income statements by using the What-If and Solver modules in Excel.[6] The model can be built in a matter of minutes and constantly adjusted before equipment is purchased and following a purchase. It is relatively accurate and, if you take a conservative approach, you can easily see the advantage of modeling and what a great help this is to decision-making.

I generally perform these on an accrual basis and then update with a cash basis to see how close my plans were. If the model shows a marginal predicted profit, I decide against the purchase. It is important to factor in trends and look carefully at replacement or the "bloom off the flower" syndrome, where the equipment appears to be the product of a fad rather than a legitimate tool with long-term usefulness. I also am resistant to the "loss-leader" concept, where the equipment is touted for its potential to produce secondary income. This may be true in some cases, but is most often the exception.

LEADERSHIP

The word *leadership* often evokes an uncomfortable twinge in the veterinarian's mind. As mentioned before, all doctors and professionals consciously or subconsciously consider themselves leaders by virtue of their position in society. They tend to think: "I'm smart and everybody likes me. I'm a natural-born leader."

In most corporations, leaders emerge out of a structure with defined requirements and specific definitions for leadership. By contrast, leaders in a typical veterinary business rise to the top by default. Most become leaders because of an unavoidable need to fill a vacuum or because of limited ownership. That vacuum can be a small or a big sucking whirlpool. Failure to perform leadership tasks and lack of respect often lead to major dysfunction in the corporation in spite of an outward appearance of compatibility. Lack of leadership and structure leads to divisive attitudes, triangulation, constant distracting chatter, tremendous wastes of energy, and, ultimately, loss of profit and quality of care. The default leader is often a senior partner or owner who, by virtue of his or her availability, is deemed the "boss." In another scenario, another partner may be designated as the chief executive officer while he remains the victim of the alpha dog and his followers. Few if any practice leaders come with real corporate experience and training.

Management and leadership is a full-time job with a multifaceted practice. The number of employees may be from 20 to more than 100. The hours devoted to this job are often greater than those of the major providers and the emotional stress can be overwhelming. The managing partner forced to put his clinical duties on hold or relegate them to other partners and employees will most likely never recover that role in the same capacity. More importantly, the managing partner will be relegated to a life-long devotion and pursuit of corporate vision. Many authors in this book have experienced this and subsequently developed great knowledge and respect for the paradigms of business. Strategic planning, Porter's principles, and many guidelines are not just fads but necessities for success and even survival.

PETER DRUCKER STATED

Management is doing things right. Leadership is doing the right things. An effective leader is not someone who is loved or admired. He or she is someone whose followers do the right thing. Popularity is not leadership. Results are.[7]

Leadership, Basic Goals, and Qualities of a Good Leader

While the external mission statement of all veterinary practices is somehow related to the health care of the horse, the internal mission statement is often based on a form of return on investment or return to the stockholders. Managers and leaders of these organizations must be determined to fulfill both the internal and external missions. The overwhelming task of the leader, however, must reach beyond these goals. The leader must also have a vision. Without a vision for the firm and its employees and a personal vision for themselves, leaders are not necessary. Then only managers are needed and an organization with only managers is doomed to stagnation and failure. The long-held concept that, if we just work hard caring for horses, the company will take care of itself, is no longer viable at any level from the small practice to the large hospital to the university and teaching institutions.

Vision does not simply involve pie-in-the-sky mission statements, but also requires a comprehensive overview and an examination of the structure of the organization. There should be a real sense of goals and accomplishment throughout the organization.

Trust, Motivation, and Vulnerability

The leader of the organization must motivate others to recognize the vision and drive for the goals. To accomplish this, the leader must develop a true feeling of trust, a difficult task. The first rule of trust is to admit vulnerability. The second rule is to be a model for others.

Kathryn Jeffers from the University of Wisconsin School of Business stated that one of the cardinal rules of leadership is to admit your mistakes the moment they are recognized: "You make a mistake, you own it, you're busted." Vulnerability is a difficult task for many people. However, hiding mistakes and failures only creates a political task that puts others and the company in harm's way. A true leader learns from his mistakes and makes an effort to move forward. He or she should create the same feeling throughout the company.

Motivation leads to a feeling of accomplishment by the employees. If they feel that you are willing to admit your mistakes and move forward, they will trust you and they will not be afraid to make suggestions to or to take risks in an attempt to realize the common vision. Admitting mistakes is not as simple as saying "I'm sorry." Often these carry painful consequences to others and yourself, particularly when they involve the painful task of dismissing an employee. This can be one of the most difficult tasks of management and leadership and can be one of the major causes of responsibility avoidance (Personal notes, Leadership Beyond Management, University of Wisconsin-Madison Executive Education, School of Business, January 2007).

Structure an Organizational Alignment

The way a veterinary practice is organized (management, departments, work teams, tasks, client processing) and the way work flows through the firm are a reflection of its structure. Alignment is the way the practice strategically operates.

Most of the characteristics of a practice's structure and alignment evolve through simple concepts derived from habit and ease of comfort: "This is the way we'll do it! I have been doing it for years and it works for me"; "We did it this way at the university, so it must be the only proper way to care for the animals." Should we make our structural plans by starting at the top with management or should we start at the bottom with staff? Most often, when groups are formed, key, loyal, and trusted individuals are added to the group because of past relationships whether they came from merging practices or from the same organization that suddenly expanded to a hospital or central organization formed by buy-in or exit strategy. The result is often a recipe for inefficiency, missed revenue, and dysfunction. The structure of the practice should be well thought out with staff aligned properly.

How do we decide on structure? Corporate notes and agreements always override the structure and are necessary from a legal standpoint. However, the real structure of the organization is tantamount to achieving the mission and goals and, in most successful practices, it centers on maximizing patient processing and cash flow. All elements of the practice are influenced by this structure and process. The framework must be strong, efficient, and enfranchised by the entire organization.

The internal structure depends on the efficiency of client processing from the original contact through patient diagnosis and care to discharge and follow-up. Information must be easily input and retrieved. Significant data must be stored and sorted for capitalization, decision-making, and marketing. The assigning of tasks should be clear to the entire staff (through job descriptions and consistent with the business vision). Regular accountability should be built into the structure (Balanced Scorecard).[8] Efficiency requires a strong overview of the tasks and an understanding of the process.

When is the patient billed? When is the surgical description recorded? Who is responsible for the discharge instructions and referral letter and what is a timely response? These tasks start and end with a well-designed computer system and depend on staff that will perform and support the practice structure.

Communication should be an important aspect of structure and be required and accounted for on a regular basis. Communication issues are often put on the back burner in a busy practice and become the number one cause for dysfunction. Strict rules should be imposed on meeting attendance. There should be rules in place for conduct and conflict. The structure of the organization should allow for a quick resolution of conflict and application of potential consequences. This is extremely difficult and remains one of the most challenging tasks of organizational alignment. Rules for regular communication help avoid and resolve conflict.

Veterinarians are technologically oriented. They are trained and disciplined to think scientifically and readily absorb, sort, and implement massive amounts of professional information, as long as it relates to their passion of improving the physical well-being of the horse and pleasing their clients. If they hope to maximize these capabilities and balance their lifestyle accordingly, then similar attention and passion will be necessary to implement and maintain the structure of a multifaceted equine practice.

CULTURE

The culture of an organization is defined as: "The dominant values, beliefs, and norms that develop over time and become relatively enduring features of organizational life."[8]

A visit to many large practices often produces an impression of personality or culture, whether it is a culture of neatness (the practice with everything bright, new, and clean), technology (the latest in everything), lifestyle (everyone is an athlete), or country doctor. Regardless, all tend to have unique characteristics that reflect their culture. However, in spite of the outward appearance, the culture may be mired in a reactive environment that resists real change and development of the practice and that suppresses vision. The skills and knowledge may be superior. However, efficiency, morale, growth, and financial success may be lacking because of the underlying culture. This again is often the result of a leadership void, poor communication, an ill-defined vision, or inherent dysfunction not due to the systems but the people responsible for its implementation. Einstein said: "People, who resist change, just continue to make the same lifelong mistakes." While each of the practices you visit may have positive cultural characteristics that create vision, many have other issues that seem to mire the organization hopelessly in the past.

Several years after the establishment of our firm, I would routinely visit the hospital on Sunday mornings after treatments were entered and gather all the inpatient records and review them for the daily charges that, at that time, were kept on a charge sheet in the back of the record. We had a system similar to most where these sheets were gathered by the front office and entered into the patient's computerized record. It was common to find $10,000 to $20,0000 of unbilled services during these sessions. I would have regular meetings with veterinary and management staff in an effort to correct these mistakes that directly erode the bottom line. At times, I could see some slight improvement but no significant change. The inability to correct this problem was in part due to structural faults and in part due to the practice culture ("This can't be happening, therefore it doesn't exist and it would take too much effort on my part to fix it"). He's the owner and it's his money and not mine. After coming to this realization I posed the question to the hospital breakout group session for several years at our early American Association of Equine Practitioners Management

Seminars. The response was amazing. Everyone felt that their way of billing (eg, white boards, night clerks) was better than mine and no one seemed to believe that it was a real problem in their practice. That was easily 10 to 15 years ago and nothing has changed. The "white board" and billing sheet still exists in most hospitals along with paper records that may or may not find their way to a permanent filing system and that are often devoid of important detailed accounting of a horse's medical record.

The right decisions are not always the most popular. When it was suggested that our company go paperless, there was a great deal of resistance. After I personally lobbied for a year for the concept, several of my office staff came to me with a solid plan to move into the system within 2 weeks. They made it clear that we were moving forward and there would be no turning back. After 2 weeks of intensive staff training, the button was pushed. All were required to comply. The younger generation was enthusiastic; the change enfranchised the entire staff to the business process, a process that only a few participated in before the change. They were amazingly competent. Only the established doctors in the practice were resistant. However, it was a short time before they realized that this process greatly freed their time, increased production, and improved service quality. Within a week, it was completely evident that the old system was forgotten. This produced a decisive change in the "culture" and resulted in an immediate and substantial increase in revenue by eliminating lost charges, greatly improving the moral of the staff, and bringing about more efficient treatment and recordkeeping.

The culture had changed from one of "can't do" to "can do" and resulted in a staff that remains proactive toward systemic innovation as well as toward more advanced technology and more efficient structure. Similar changes have been made with departmentalization of profit centers and cost of goods sales and inventory management. The cost of goods management had consistently shown a frustrating loss with reports showing the same items as the core of the problem. Our staff enthusiastically approached the issue as a challenge and devised a number of improvements in the system in an attempt to minimize the loss. They are independently seeking newer technology and devising checks and balances that do not tax the system. It continues to improve. Again, when I approach colleagues with these facts, I am greeted with disbelief and denial. You can only come to this realization through change and a solid cost of goods system. The culture must change first. While this applies to all practices, it is a necessity for survival in a multifaceted practice in the future marketplace.

If business development is not part of the individual behavior, then you will likely not see development. Cultural changes can occur in spite of resistance from the principles. However, it will take a great deal of leadership, coaching, and mentoring, even if it sometimes comes from the consensus of your staff as with our change to a paperless environment.

FINAL THOUGHTS

There is no simple recipe for designing a multifaceted practice. As mentioned, volumes have been written that go far beyond the scope of this publication. However, key to any design is the devotion of the people involved and the proper positioning of such people in the organization. Anyone designing such a practice also must pay keen attention to details and a keep a finger constantly on the pulse of the business from a visionary and financial stance. As practices grow, profits are realized from savings or scrutinizing financials. However, larger profits are derived mainly through building additional sales, pursuing a clear vision, and making shrewd investments. Like for every small business, success in the multifaceted practice is clearly tied to such factors as applying financial acumen, using forward thinking, choosing the right technology, accommodating a desirable lifestyle, maintaining a vision, and having a willingness to take a calculated risk.

REFERENCES

1. Bryant A. New York Times, May 24, 2009;1 BU.
2. Robert P. Magnus. Equine business management strategies. Oconomowoc (WI) Available at: www.equinebusinessmanagement.com. Oconomowoc (WI).
3. Vetstar, Advanced Technology, Corp. Ramsey (NJ), Available at: www.vetstar.com.
4. Lyons Kelly. The one percent difference: small change—big impact. AuthorHouse.
5. Carlberg Conrad. Business analysis with Microsoft Excel. 3rd edition. Que; 2007. Chapter 12.
6. Solver add-in: Microsoft Excel. 2007.
7. Hesselbein F, Goldsmith M, Beckhard R. The leaders of the future. San Francisco (CA): Jossey-Bass; 1996.
8. Aquila AJ, Rice CL. Compensation as a strategic asset, the new paradigm. AICPA; 2007. Chapter 5.

Design of an Equine Ambulatory Practice

F. Richard Lesser, DVM[a], R. Reynolds Cowles, Jr, DVM[b]

KEYWORDS

- Porters 5 forces • Customer service • Respect
- Fees • Change

In the past, the standard model for starting an ambulatory practice was defining an area, setting up a vehicle, establishing a telephone number, retaining an answering service or machine, and going out to promote our services at local equine events and gatherings. Practitioners depended on word of mouth, stamina, charm, and the goodwill of their friends. Veterinarians worked long hours and did just fine financially, but one might have reason to question the subsequent lifestyle.

Although that method of hope and hard work has succeeded for many in the past, there is no denying that the model of equine practice has changed. Group practices now outnumber single practitioners. This has allowed for sharing of on-call duties, equipment, and complimentary skill sets to augment services. The number of hours worked by a veterinarian each week has dropped from an exhaustive and unhealthy high of 80 hours to a more sensible and pleasant 40 to 45 hours. Many younger veterinarians expect to work even less hours, because many men and women currently in practice value a better quality of life. Clients have switched from a demand for goods to a demand for services (they can and do buy their dewormers on the Internet). The level of practice (in terms of technology and skills) has been raised to an all-time high, giving even the most modest practices a greater sense of professional satisfaction. Clients are bombarded with "expert opinions" from all sides, yet still view the quality veterinary practice as the most valued source of information and service for the health needs of their horses. Capital investment, overhead costs, and salary expectations have skyrocketed, and successful practices have learned to manage their practices in a proactive fashion The days of simply showing up and working hard are gone forever. Today's practitioners must actively manage so that their resources can be leveraged in such a fashion that a return can be realized on their capital investment and the hours spent in practice. These changes are all for the better. We are privileged to practice here and now, when there has never been a more exciting or rewarding time to attend to the welfare of the horse.

[a] The Equine Clinic at OakenCroft, 880 Bridge Street, Ravena, NY 12143, USA
[b] Blue Ridge Equine Clinic, Earlysville, VA, USA
E-mail address: ecolesser@aol.com (F.R. Lesser); ecolesser@aol.com (R.R. Cowles).

Vet Clin Equine 25 (2009) 489–498
doi:10.1016/j.cveq.2009.07.007
0749-0739/09/$ – see front matter © 2009 Elsevier Inc. All rights reserved.

The author suggests a more systematic approach to the design of an ambulatory practice that should answer the needs of group and solo practices. In setting up or rejuvenating an ambulatory practice, one must first decide on a geographic area and an emphasis on general equine work, performance horses, broodmares, or the race track. Each of these areas dictates the overall design. It would be helpful for the practitioner to have previous familiarity with the location and a working knowledge of the segment of the horse industry to be served. Horse owners are more accepting of a veterinarian who understands their specific problems and needs. Satisfied veterinarians want to work with animals and owners they understand and enjoy. It can and should be a win-win situation.

There is a general business model that applies to equine veterinary practices that considers the forces all practices must respond to. That model is called "Porter's Five Forces" and was designed by Michael Porter of the Harvard Business School.[1] These five forces are incoming, outgoing, internal, environmental, and global. The author reviews these forces as they apply to ambulatory practice because they form a logical setup of a practice.

How one attracts and handles requests for services (incoming forces) is critical to the success of a practice. In the author's experience, most horse owners want to talk to a person. That person is the most important person in the practice other than the veterinarian. His or her voice must be warm and compassionate, knowledgeable, able to convey information accurately, and able to instill a confidence in the client that his or her message is going to be transmitted to the veterinarian and that it is going to be acted on in a timely fashion. A well-managed practice cultivates and nurtures not just the receptionist but all the lay staff that contact these incoming forces.

Be aware that the motivation of lay staff members to perform their duties well is often not solely for financial rewards. They are often motivated by a concern for the patients, dedication to the practice, and bonds with the clients. Many of them have been with the practice for longer than some of the veterinary staff, and the clients see them as a source of continuity. The office manager is the person with the answers. The receptionist who consistently answers their calls is viewed as the familiar advocate for their horse health concerns. The bookkeeper who justly deals with billing situations is considered to be honest and precise. The technicians and assistants are the people who care for their horses compassionately and tirelessly. For those practices with even the most modest haul-in facilities, the barn workers are the ones who keep the place clean and help clients to back their trailers and load their horses. The clients quickly come to view them as a defining part of the practice. If you have a small practice with a single person wearing all those hats (and doing so with style), you need to treat that person as the most valuable asset your practice has.

It is well accepted that friendly competent office staff have a monumental effect on the success of the practice. At the same time, rude, lazy, and sullen folks are poison. If the staff members enjoy a good relationship with you, they are going to be quick to go the extra distance for you. If they have confidence that you are talented and hardworking, they are going to be sure the clients see things that way as well. Conversely, if you leave the staff feeling abused and misused, the clients are likely to hear it in their tone that you are less than stellar.

It is really quite simple. Do as you promise. Keep communications open and your staff informed of your schedule. Treat them fairly, honestly, and respectfully. Never leave employees in a no-win situation. Pay them well, and expect them to perform for that pay. Periodic reviews not only address performance but serve as a means of development. The new expanded model of ambulatory practice brings a need for human resource management that must be addressed. As a manager, there is no

public accountant (CPA) management firms offer office training that has application in equine practices.[3] The AAEP summer practice management seminar offers a wide range of educational opportunities custom-built by equine veterinarians for equine veterinary practices. Often, good service-oriented employees can be found outside the equine or veterinary field. Their desire to provide service and skill sets can minimize their temporary lack of horse knowledge. It may be easier to teach them our vocabulary than to teach a gifted horse owner about business communications and organization.

Managing employees, facilities, inventories, and equipment becomes exponentially more important as a practice grows. The one doctor–one assistant practice may have minimal issues that can be managed easily with simple job lists and employment agreements. Larger practices may find it beneficial to have a more systematic approach in place that may involve procedure and policy manuals for a whole range of management and human resource issues (eg, contracts, job descriptions, performance policies, annual reviews, health care benefits, rights to veterinary goods and services, harassment prevention protocols, drug use, time off, continuing education, appearance, ethics, confidentiality, equipment maintenance, marketing, accounting, mentoring, strategic planning, inventory, computer systems, vehicle logs, controlled drugs).

Such a list may seem overwhelming, but for the growing practice, trying to react to these situations after the fact is monumentally more difficult and less successful than managing them from a proactive position would have been. Some veterinarians may determine that they have no desire to deal with these potential challenges and that they would rather just practice the art and science of veterinary medicine. In that case, you would be well advised to remain an employee or a sole owner without any significant management responsibilities. Alternatively, in a larger practice, you could recognize that your strength lies practicing rather than managing and that you should hire a capable manager. As an ambulatory practice grows past three to four members, it becomes abundantly apparent that someone, be that person a veterinarian or an office manager, must have an understanding of the vision and mission of the practice and be available on a regular basis to steer the practice along that path. Practices that have ignored this advice often implode because of a lack of dedicated management.

In the real world, many beginning practices have done well by having a few people, often family members, with a shared vision wearing multiple hats (receptionist, billing, horse handling, computer entry, bookkeeping, client communication, and veterinary services). Even these small models need to have well-defined lines of communication and responsibilities to prevent conflicting and confusing voices being heard by the employees. This need increases as the number of employees increases. Often, family members dictating business and professional decisions to associates and partners may lead to unrest within the practice and stress inside the family. If so, once a practice can afford outside staffing, it is advisable to move family members out of the business structure.

Some ambulatory practitioners value their "quiet time" between calls. Others welcome the company of an assistant who can hold horses, enter computer data, interact with clients, field and return telephone calls, move equipment, prepare injection sites, assist with procedures, and stock vehicles. Such an assistant can greatly increase efficiency and profitability in practices, which leverages them beyond the status of merely driving and companionability.

Practice management software and computer systems not only influence the outgoing forces but are now the common thread that ties together all your internal forces. There are many choices of management software and hardware, but it is the opinion of the author that each has strong points and weaknesses and there is no one clearly superior system available today. There are several identifiable characteristics that you may want to consider before investing in a system. Topping that list is the stability and reliability of the software vendor. Unfortunately, many vendors have entered and left the market without providing continuing support for their systems. A software provider with a significant share of the market that is also willing to connect you with established practices that use the provider's product would carry less risk. Technical support should have a reputation of being accessible and responsive. Many ambulatory practices have seen the benefits of remote processing, only to find that there are technical issues with uploading the mobile units to the clinic database.

You may want to identify the hidden costs of your system. Mandatory upgrades, re-licensing fees, support levels, and additional hardware required by upgrades can add significant costs to the system you buy. Your system must make intuitive sense to you and be simple to use. It should cover all your medical record needs and generate management reports that you find useful. The speed of the system and the ease of data entry are not uniform across companies, so be sure to compare systems before buying. Younger practices may want a system that can economically and reliably expand instead of being discarded and replaced with another system that requires expensive data transfer and retraining.

Systems that create an invoice automatically as you create a medical record are superior because they do a better job of capturing fees than does simple invoicing alone. It is also important that your system readily communicate with other electronic data you use (eg, Internet, messaging and scheduling modules, image archiving, electronic Coggin's and health certificates, laboratory, inventory, credit card processing, accounting).

An accountant is a universal recommendation for even smaller practices, and that person usually has definite recommendations for the financial software systems that he or she is comfortable in working with. Any accounting software that you choose should use a chart of accounts that addresses your needs as an equine practitioner. The *Equine Veterinary Practice Chart of Accounts* has recently been compiled by Dr Marsha L. Heinke.[4] This resource is made available to practitioners by industry leaders Milburn, Webster, and Pfizer.

Smaller practices may find it cost-effective and simple to provide payroll services in-house. As the practice grows, outsourcing this service becomes much simpler and more economic.

Quality practices are only possible when they charge and collect fees that are appropriate for the services rendered. Historically, equine practice has not maintained a fee schedule adequate to cover expenses and salaries and to provide a return on investment. In the past decade, this situation created a crisis situation for equine practitioners, who could no longer attract and retain associates or partners. In more recent years, management consultants and management groups have led the battle to charge appropriate fees, and we have witnessed a healthy resurgence among our colleagues.

In determining a fee structure, it is possible to begin by comparing your fees with a regional database of historical fees. This should not be confused with "fee setting," wherein neighbors band together to create a uniform fee schedule. Such action is neither legal nor ethical. The National Commission on Veterinary Economic Issues (NCVEI) maintains a free interactive Web site resource[5] providing historical benchmarking data for fees that is helpful. Benchmarking should be viewed only as a starting point for determining your fees, however, and the final fee structure should reflect your costs and expected returns for every item you invoice. Many practices have been able to create their own fee schedules, whereas others have wisely turned to practice consultants and software vendors for guidance.

Equally important to generating fees is collecting them. Many practices of all sizes have shifted to a policy for payment at the time of service, including the widespread use of credit cards for absentee owners. A written credit policy is mandatory for any practice, but just like any other written policy, it is useless unless it is strictly followed. A starting practice is actually better poised to deal with accounts receivable than is an established practice. It can be hard to explain to a client who has always been given 60 to 90 days to pay a bill why he or she can no longer do so. It is much simpler just to make it an initial policy that payment is expected at the time of service.

Most absentee owners should have a credit card that can be preapproved for payment of their accounts. A client with no credit card but who wishes to have what is, in effect, a limitless line of credit with you should raise a red flag. If a financial institution that is an expert in the field of credit has denied someone a card, it would be a foolhardy veterinarian, whose strength is medicine rather than finance, to offer it instead. Be aware that there is considerable liability in keeping client credit card numbers "on file" in your office. A better and more secure system would use remote storage of the credit card information with the processing company that you use.

Always remember that owning horses is not a right but a privilege, and with privilege comes responsibility. Do not let clients make their horses your problem. The owner's responsibility is to contract for his or her animals' heath care, and the veterinarian is responsible for fulfilling that contract. Do not let them tell you that you are less than compassionate or even selfish when requiring them to pay for your services.

It is the commendable nature of the people who enter this profession to be compassionate, but be aware that you can only give what you have. In a single-person practice, any goods or services that you give away affect your bottom line. In a multiple-person practice with even a small lay staff, any pro bono work cuts directly into your ability to attract and retain quality help. Anything that your employed veterinarians and lay staff provide for free is, in effect, money out of your family budget. You may find it useful to set a policy of billing for every item and service that you provide and then to itemize "compassion discounts" or "courtesy discounts" on your invoices when your sense of compassion impels you.

Management of accounts receivable (AR) is no fun, but it is even less enjoyable to work hard and have nothing to show for it. To manage your AR, you need to track them and then routinely review the outstanding accounts and implement collection actions when needed. One useful method of determining AR is to calculate how long after you provide a service you are paid for it. This calculation, referred to as "days on the books," should be less than 30 days for a healthy equine practice.

$$\text{Days on the Books} = \text{Total Accounts Receivable}$$
$$\div \ (\text{past 12 months gross}/365 \text{ days})$$

As an example, a practice grossing \$300,000 has outstanding accounts of \$30,000.

$$\text{Days on the Books} = \$30,000 \div (\$30,000/365 \text{ days}) = 36.5 \text{ Days}$$

Practices of every size can benefit from some management help in defining, tracking, and managing the internal forces that exist in your practice. The first necessity is to create a team that includes an accountant, lawyer, and banker who are familiar with (or willing to learn about) equine ambulatory veterinary practices and enlist their services. Local firms may meet your needs, but there are also several national practice management specialists who offer services that extend beyond simple tax planning and preparation.

The NCVEI not only has a means of benchmarking your fees but is especially valuable to smaller ambulatory practices in that it provides comprehensive industry standards and insights in many areas of practice (eg, pricing, finance, operations, products and services, human resources, and marketing). This resource is a free benefit provided by membership in the American Veterinary Medical Association (AVMA) and is time-efficient, especially for the single practitioner who may be hard pressed to justify time away from the practice engaged in more intense management venues.

These other resources are only valuable insofar as the practice is dedicated to acting on them. Hiring a consultant who generates an incisive and insightful (and costly) analysis of your practice is only helpful if you are ready, willing, and eager to act on the findings. The same goes for enrollment in veterinary management or study groups.[6] These gatherings are ongoing intense multiple-day sessions covering all aspects of practice management with a recurring group of similar practices over many years (see resources for contact information).

The environmental forces affecting a practice are defined as external forces beyond your control. These may include licensing, zoning laws, state board requirements, horse density, changes in the horse industry in your area, and the influence other practices in the area have on you. Before deciding on a geographic location, one should research these forces to be sure that your proposed market and business plan are, in fact, viable.

The typical equine ambulatory practice has much lower overhead in terms of facilities and staffing than exists for clinics and hospitals, but this plus is often negated by long nonproductive hours spent driving from farm to farm. Technology is helpful in defining the shortest route from point A to point B. Several economic mapping systems can arrange a whole schedule of calls in the most efficient fashion and simultaneously determine your travel times, enabling you to manage your schedule and set your fees accordingly.

The presence of an assistant may allow you to organize your day better, because that person provides help that, otherwise, the owner could only have provided at times that would be less efficient for you. Calls can be grouped in certain regions for particular days of the week to increase efficiency, and thus keep farm visit fees reasonable. For those calls that come in from outside the defined area and cannot wait, it is realistic to charge a higher fee to cover your higher costs.

Some practices have successfully reduced driving time by organizing regional haul-in centers that result in greater efficiency for the practice and lower costs for the owners. Many ambulatory practices maintain modest haul-in facilities for well-horse visits and lameness diagnostics. By keeping these facilities streamlined, they can increase efficiency without adding to the enormous cost in terms of manpower, equipment, and supplies that comes along with hospital cases.

Practice vehicles carry significant accounting responsibilities to comply with Internal Revenue Service (IRS) rules. There is a fine balance to be struck between economic gas mileage, purchase price, repairs, and durability. Good-quality, low-mileage, used vehicles may be good investments for many practices considering the number of miles that are going to be placed on them during their use. Vehicle leases, although deductible, may not be economic, because the level of miles that ambulatory practices accrue may result in large fees for over-limit mileage. Your vehicle may also have a potential to have a negative impact on your practice marketing if it is judged by your clients to be too expensive (Doc must be raking it in to get a new $75,000 luxury sport utility vehicle every year) or too amateurish (can't see how that junker gets from farm to farm). No matter what you drive, be sure it is clean and professional looking. A careful analysis of costs (including professional time spent driving and fluctuations in fuel prices) is needed to determine farm fees. Because farm call fees may be inelastic and are often "shopped" by clients, some practices have Increased their prices for professional service (which are more elastic) slightly to cover the lower farm call fees they need to be competitive.

Successful ambulatory practices anticipate changes in the local horse industry and are flexible enough to retool, restaff, and retrain to meet the changing needs in their market. Loss of open pasture land may drive out broodmare practices, but these areas often have growing performance horse populations owned by the new residents. The downturn in racing has affected track practitioners and those working on broodmares and sales horses, motivating many of those practitioners to reinvent their practices.

It is important to keep open lines of communication and maintain good relationships with colleagues, even in competitive areas. Collegiality usually results in better practice for all and good sound economics. Those who engage in fee cutting and speaking ill of others usually do not succeed, and those who take an ethical approach usually prosper. It is often said that the place to open a new practice is where the horse owner is used to good-quality veterinary service by competent practitioners.

The global factors include national economic trends, tax law, and the number and quality of new graduates being turned out by our schools, for example. These factors are often outside of any given individual's control, but an awareness of and engagement with them gives a practice manager a distinct advantage over the long haul. The civic-minded practitioner is informed of and invested in the decisions that affect our communities and our profession. Involvement in local planning boards, business groups, racing authorities, veterinary colleges, and state and national organizations is the mark of a visionary manager. Only those who are actively involved can make changes and have the right to complain about the state of affairs. The others are just along for the ride.

Ambulatory practice has the potential to reward those proactively engaged in it in professional and financial terms. It also has the capability of creating a life of misery for those who do not develop a culture of excellence in their personal and professional lives. Dr Lyle Sussman (Chairman and Professor of Management, College of Business and Public Administration, University of Louisville) has shared with the AAEP a simple law that applies not only to ambulatory practice but to life in general. Sussman's law states that we all get exactly what we deserve in life.[7] If your research indicates a need for your kind of veterinarian in your proposed locality; you have good skills, professionalism, and a dedication to lifelong learning; you have a vision and dedication to your mission and the welfare of the horse; you design a practice that meets the service needs of your clients; you invest time and resources into managing that practice; you treat your clients, employees, and colleagues with justice and respect; you maintain fair charges and collect the money in a timely fashion; and you find fulfillment in your professional, civic, and person life, then you are likely to succeed and you deserve it. Conversely, if your practice has no planning, no goals, no respect or sense of justice, inadequate fees, poor collegial relationships with neighbors, indifference or disdain of your employees, and no sense of place in the world, you are likely to fail miserably and you deserve it. The difference in these two scenarios is stark. The authority to choose one over the other lies within you.

REFERENCES

1. Porter ME. Competitive strategy: techniques for analyzing industries and competitors. New York: The Free Press; 1980.
2. Covey SR. The 7 habits of highly effective people. New York: Fireside; 1989.
3. Heinke ML, McCarthy JB. Practice made perfect: a guide to veterinary practice management. Lakewood: AAHA Press; 2001.
4. Heinke ML. Equine veterinary practice chart of accounts. Phoenix (AZ): Milburn Equine; 2006.
5. Available at: http://www.ncvei.org. Accessed February, 2009.
6. Veterinary Study Groups, Inc. Available at: http://www.veterinarystudygroups.com. Accessed February 28, 2009.
7. Sussman L. Solving the people puzzle. In: Proceedings of the AAEP Practice Management Seminar, Lexington, KY, July 25, 1999.

Medical Records in Equine Veterinary Practice

Susan H. Werner, BA[a,b]

KEYWORDS

- Medical records • Equine • Practice management
- Practice workflow • Risk management

Quality medical records are the cornerstone of successful equine veterinary practice. The scope and integrity of the information contained in a practice's medical records influence the quality of patient care and client service and affect liability risk, practice productivity, and overall practice value.

How do we define medical records? What is the historical perspective regarding medical records? What information should a medical record contain? What are the basic tasks associated with medical records? What opportunities exist in daily workflow for gathering information? What methods can we use to enter information? What important issues affect medical records in equine practice? How can we create high-quality records? What are the lasting benefits of quality medical records for an equine practice?

The dynamic nature of equine veterinary practice means that our needs regarding medical records also continually change. To stay successful, we must regularly reassess medical records requirements and consider new strategies, processes, and resources that can enable us to meet our needs now and in the future.

MEDICAL RECORDS: A DEFINITION

Medical records are organized accounts of all patient care-related information created or received by a practice. They can be a physical paper file containing documents and materials, an electronic database of patient-related information, or images, for example, in varying formats or a combination of a paper file and electronic database. Practices use medical records to record patient-related encounters and history, facilitate patient care, communicate with clients and other caregivers, produce reports of information, teach, and generate research data.

[a] Werner Equine, LLC, 20 Godard Road, PO Box 5, North Granby, CT 06060, USA
[b] RxWorks, Inc, 6375 S Pecos Road, Street 202, Las Vegas, NV 89120, USA
E-mail address: susan@wernerequine.com

Vet Clin Equine 25 (2009) 499–510
doi:10.1016/j.cveq.2009.07.010
0749-0739/09/$ – see front matter © 2009 Elsevier Inc. All rights reserved.

vetequine.theclinics.com

HISTORICAL PERSPECTIVE: HOW HAVE MEDICAL RECORDS CHANGED?

Each type of equine practice (eg, smaller private practices, referral clinics, academia, reproduction, racetrack, industry) has its own unique needs regarding medical records. Therefore, the methods of gathering information, formats for entering data, and requirements for access to records and reporting differ.

We now view older systems of manually entering information repetitively into message books, notes, or forms as too time-consuming and paper dependent. Previously, patient folders were jammed with travel or work sheets, invoices, statements, laboratory test results, radiographic films, reports, and letters, for example. Entering brief summaries of patient care by means of free text on paper after patient visits relied on the provider's ability to recall every service and medication provided. Because few people remembered every detail, this process often led to incomplete and inaccurate records.

Access to previous history at a new visit or consultation meant retrieving the correct patient folder and sorting through papers to find the specific information needed. Plagued by problems of illegibility, lost or misplaced files, cryptic abbreviations, and incomplete information, this outdated system impaired efficient cost-effective delivery of appropriate care. Dictation and transcription only increased the number of people involved in the process, tape quality was often unreliable, and significant room for error remained. Practices were vulnerable if malpractice threats arose and accurate and comprehensive records were not readily available.

Today, changing standards of care, innovations in scientific and information technologies, amplified consumer demand for information, and increased liability risk continue to have an impact on medical records. Zoonotic disease considerations are changing practice communications, protocols, reporting requirements, and record content. Any type of communications (eg, verbal, written, electronic) with horse owners, agents, or handlers about cases that might involve zoonotic disease should be carefully documented. Diagnostic and treatment services for such cases must be detailed in the medical record. Experts versed in malpractice matters report that "Veterinarians are becoming increasingly viewed as protectors of general public health and with that responsibility has come increasing numbers of malpractice disputes."[1] Effective protocols educating staff members about how to handle such cases, good communications, and comprehensive medical records can minimize such liability risks.

New methods of communication are constantly emerging. We can now use e-mail and text messages to send reminders and recalls. E-mail consultations are commonplace. Like their human counterparts, some veterinary practices now offer client portals on their Web sites. Using a secure Internet connection, owners can pay a bill or access medical record information online. Human medicine and veterinary medicine are exploring the use of Web-based repositories of medical record information. The repositories could allow animal owners to access and manage information on sites outside of the practices in which their animals are treated. Information is portable and controlled by the patient's owner instead of each practice. These new opportunities bring different challenges for practice owners and managers as they evaluate communications, recordkeeping, and security needs.

In most practices, information technology (IT) has revolutionized medical records and reduced many of the risks created by the older paper-based systems. Electronic medical records (EMRs) have dramatically improved our ability to enter, organize, store, and retrieve information quickly. Streamlined electronic data entry makes building problem-oriented medical records much less complicated. We can enter data directly into the record at the time of service with minimal effort. Patient history is readily available stall-side to facilitate better care. Users can simultaneously generate a medical record entry and correlated billing charges.

WHAT INFORMATION SHOULD A MEDICAL RECORD CONTAIN?

Regulatory and statute requirements for content of medical records vary from state to state in the United States and among countries. Practices should consult the requirements published by the various jurisdictions in which they are located. It is also important to remember that "A veterinarian licensed in multiple states is bound by the laws of each of those states and the federal government."[2] The American Veterinary Medical Association (AVMA), American Association of Equine Practitioners (AAEP), and other organizations have standards and guidelines regarding medical records that are available through their Web sites and publications.

Most lists of content requirements include the following categories:

- Patient information
- Owner information
- Patient encounter or visit information
- Information received during daily practice workflow

The author has included several entries that she has found important to record during more than 30 years of managing an equine practice. Medical records should include but are not limited to the following entries.

Patient Information

- Patient signalment or identification, including species, age and date of birth, breed, gender, color, markings, registration and microchip numbers, brands, tattoos, and the practice's unique identification number, for example
- Other relevant patient care-related information, such as location, trainers, caregivers, and farriers, for example
- Insurance providers
- Patient history (eg, medical, surgical, vaccination, reproductive, dental, parasite control, behavioral, physical environment)
- Previous problems, diagnostics, treatment, patient response, and resolution
- Current problems, medications, diet, supplements, and therapies
- Special farriery requirements, shoeing, or therapies

Owner Information

- Name and practice's unique identification number
- Authorized agents
- Address and means of contact (eg, telephone numbers, e-mail addresses, physical addresses)
- Referring parties or practices

Patient Encounter or Visit Information

At initial contact with practice (to veterinarian, answering service, or staff member)

- Author of medical record entry
- Date, time, place, and method of initial contact
- Identification of person contacting practice

- If person is not the owner or designated agent, description of efforts made to reach the owner or agent
- Presenting complaint
- Patient history provided
- Any other pertinent patient- or visit-related information provided or reviewed
- Outcome of contact: scheduled or emergency visit and visit arrangement details
- Signed forms (eg, veterinary care plan [estimate], informed consent forms, registration forms, releases)

At patient visit (in chronologic order, with author identified for each entry)

- Date, time, and location of visit
- Any extenuating circumstances at visit that affected patient care or the visit experience
- Notation of individuals present at visit
- Review and addendum to pertinent history
- Review of presenting complaint and problems
- General observations of patient
- Pertinent examinations and findings
- Assessment: differential or definitive diagnoses when pertinent
- Plan for diagnostics or therapy
- Diagnostics, reports, and interpretation of findings (eg, laboratory testing, imaging)
- Treatments and patient response
- Medications administered, including when, by whom, product, dosage, routes, duration, rates (if applicable), frequency, and site (if applicable); if required, product batch may also be noted
- Medications dispensed or prescribed, including product, dosage, routes, duration, frequency, and site (if applicable); if required, product batch may also be noted
- Details of any general anesthesia or surgery, including surgeon identification and duration of procedure
- Prognosis, if applicable
- Reports from referring practices and consultants
- Referral information if patient is sent to a specialist or referral practice
- Aftercare instructions and any plan for follow-up visits or contacts (eg, reminders, recall, appointments)
- Progress notes
- Waivers or postponement of recommended care

After visit

- Details of reports received or solicited regarding patient progress in any format (eg, telephone, direct contact, e-mail, text message)
- Forms or reports linked to patient visit
- Recommended changes in therapy or environment, for example, conveyed by any method (eg, telephone, direct contact, e-mail, text message)
- Waiver, postponement, or failure to follow care recommendations
- Resolution of patient's problem

Information from Patient Care-Related Encounters Throughout Daily Workflow

- Owner-signed forms, including registration forms, consent forms, and authorizations to release information, for example
- Objective documentation of client complaints and resolutions
- Forms and reports generated at client or regulatory agency requests (eg, scratch forms, vaccination reports, medications reporting, health certificates)
- Recommended schedules of wellness care, including wellness examinations, vaccinations, dental care, and parasite control, for example
- Prescription refills, including time, date, product, concentration, dosage, route, frequency, and length of treatment
- Logs of direct or telephone conversations with owner or agents regarding patient care; logs should include:
  - Author of medical record entry
  - Date, time, place, and method of contact
  - Identification of person making contact
  - If person is not the owner or designated agent, description of efforts made to reach the owner or agent
  - Presenting complaint, concern, or question
  - Any pertinent patient history or information provided or reviewed
  - Outcome of contact (eg, scheduled or emergency visit, resolution of concern with no visit scheduled, patient progress report, general discussion of care, prescription refill)
- Electronic communications (eg, e-mails or telefaxes printed as portable document format [PDF] files and electronically added to the record or placed in a paper file
- Communications received by means of mail placed in paper files or scanned as PDF files and entered into the record electronically

WHAT ARE THE BASIC TASKS ASSOCIATED WITH MEDICAL RECORDS?
Setting Up the System

The first step in creating good medical records is to determine desired content (**Fig. 1**) (ie, what information you want each record to contain); how you want to enter information, organize it, and access it; and how you want to generate reports. Work with your practice IT team (in smaller practices, this might mean only the veterinarian) and your software provider's representatives.

Take time to learn what your software program can do and how you can customize it to meet your practice's needs. As you set up your system, it is critical to understand the implications of setup decisions for the different users and points of use in your practice's daily workflow. It is much more efficient to make informed setup decisions than to fix problems later.

Creating Medical Records

Staff must clearly understand what information should be noted, why they are meant to record it, and when to enter it. Ideally, data entry should be easy, intuitive, and time-saving. When entering data, staff should use Subjective, Objective, Assessment, Plan (SOAP) and History, Exam, Assessment, Plan (HEAP) formats, standardized terminology, and templates that complement free text to speed the process. The goals are to create records that are comprehensive, accurate, and easily understood by the people who read them.

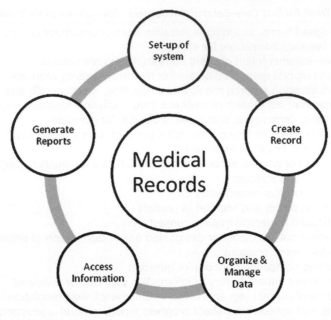

Fig. 1. Basic tasks associated with medical records. (*Courtesy of* RxWorks, Inc.)

Organizing and Managing the Records

Software can handle the organization of electronically captured data, but practices need to establish protocols for organizing and managing ancillary paper reports and materials.

Accessing Medical Records

The needs of different users (eg, veterinarian, technician, administrative staff) and point-of-use requirements are important considerations regarding access to medical records. Often, practices can customize software and organize files in ways that make access easy for the different users. It is particularly important that veterinarians have easy access to medical records at a visit so that they may access history.

Medical Record Reports

Users should be able to generate comprehensive reports from stored patient and client information. Although most software programs produce patient history and other standard reports, practices may need to create custom reports to meet other requirements. Getting data out of a system should be as easy as putting it in. Define the contents of reports you regularly use, who has access to them, and how you want to handle requests for reports.

WHAT ARE THE OPPORTUNITIES IN A PRACTICE'S WORKFLOW FOR GATHERING MEDICAL RECORD INFORMATION?

There are numerous opportunities in practice workflow for gathering information that belongs in the medical record. These include before the patient visit, at the patient visit, after the patient visit, and throughout the daily workflow (**Fig. 2**). Information gathering involves veterinarians, practice employees, patient owners or agents, regulatory

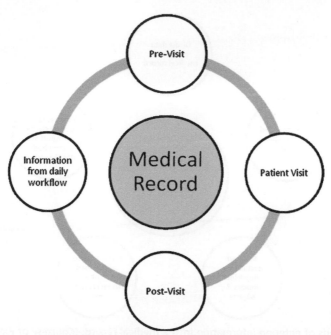

Fig. 2. Workflow opportunities for gathering medical record information. (*Courtesy of* RxWorks, Inc.)

agencies, numerous ancillary service providers, and referring or referral veterinarians, for example. Medical record creation should interface easily with a practice's daily workflow and other related tasks, such as billing.

WHAT ARE THE METHODS OF ENTERING INFORMATION INTO A MEDICAL RECORD?

Because medical records document all patient care-related information, they are an integral part of practice communications. Information exchanges can be internal (within the practice) or external (between the practice and an individual or entity outside of the practice). The methods of communicating information are verbal, text, and electronic (**Fig. 3**).

WHAT IMPORTANT ISSUES AFFECT MEDICAL RECORDS IN EQUINE PRACTICE?
Point-of-user Functionality for Your Practice

How well do the processes governing medical records in your practice work for the various users in the situations they regularly encounter in daily workflow? Can veterinarians find the information they need? Is it easy to log on and enter pertinent information? Can schedulers and admission or discharge staff find information quickly and record data easily to build comprehensive and accurate records? Can managers and owners readily generate informative reports that allow them to strategize, budget, and plan for the practice? Is it easy to track cases by diagnoses or presenting complaints for research and patient care planning?

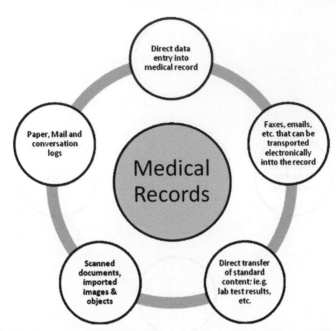

Fig. 3. Methods of entering information into a medical record. (*Courtesy of* RxWorks, Inc.)

Interoperability

"Interoperability is the ability of different IT systems and software applications to communicate, to exchange data accurately, effectively, and consistently, and to use information that has been exchanged."[3] Extending that definition, all appropriate viewers must be able to share and understand the information contained in medical records easily. To make records readily understood, practices must consider legibility (for all nonelectronic data entry), standard abbreviations and terminology, use of customized data entry templates (eg, SOAP, HEAP), and following guidelines for creating problem-oriented records. Quickly scratched notes that no one else can decipher should no longer exist.

Ethical and Legal Concerns

Please consult the *Principles of Veterinary Medical Ethics* of the AVMA[4] and the *AAEP Ethical and Professional Guidelines*[2] for detailed requirements regarding the ethical and legal aspects of medical records.

Confidentiality

"Ethically, the information within veterinary medical records is considered privileged and confidential. It must not be released except by court order or consent of the owner of the patient."[2] It is important for the practice to implement training and written protocols that can help practice employees to understand and support these requirements.

Ownership

"Medical records are the property of the practice and the practice owner. The original records must be retained by the practice for the period required by statute."[2]

Copies of Medical Records

"Veterinarians are obligated to provide copies or summaries of medical records when requested by the client. Veterinarians should secure a written release to document that request."[2] Such requests and consents also become part of the medical record.

Retention and Destruction

A practice should consult its state or regional statues and regulations for the specific requirements that apply to its practices regarding retention and destruction of records.[2]

Risk Management

Risk management experts repeatedly state, "Good medical records combined with timely client communication are important factors in reducing malpractice claims."[5] The bottom line is that excellent records can minimize several types of risk.

The availability of detailed, comprehensive, and error-free medical records is critical to defending license complaints and malpractice actions. Documentation of potentially dangerous patient behavior may also protect veterinarians, staff, handlers, and others present at a patient visit from possible injury. In some situations, recorded warnings about a patient's potentially dangerous behavior may also prevent injury to other animals.

Breaches of medical record confidentiality are also major concerns. Practices should develop and publish in-house security and privacy protocols, train staff members, and carefully follow and enforce their policies. Access to sensitive information should be physically and electronically restricted (see the section on security elsewhere in this article).

Providing a copy of your practice's privacy policy in information packets for new clients can educate and reassure your clients that you take steps to protect the information they have entrusted to you.

Some special situations in equine practice warrant extra attention and often creation of special protocol linked to medical records.[4] These situations include but are not limited to the following[5]:

- Prepurchase examinations
- Emergency visits
- Referred cases
- Patients flagged in the system as having behavior concerns that might increase risk factors for human and patient injury
- Patients involved in leases
- Insurance examinations
- Euthanasia
- Absentee owner (ie, those not present at patient visits)
- Clients who have been flagged as difficult, demanding, or angry
- Reports to nonowners containing medical record information
- Multiple-clinic practices with personnel at various locales
- Veterinary care plans (estimates)
- Cases that result in negative or unexpected outcomes
- General anesthesia and surgery
- Laminitis
- Colic
- Rectal tears
- Wounds

- Sales work
- Breeding work
- Incorporation of records from previous systems into new systems
- Records required by parimutuel jurisdictions

Appropriate insurance protection is critical to minimize risk. Practices should consult with insurance carriers and carry adequate insurance to cover the various risks associated with medical records.

Security

Practices should set and enforce appropriate protocols and security measures to restrict physical and electronic access to medical records to only those individuals possessing proper credentials.

Examples of physical access restrictions include requirements to lock computers, vehicles, and offices. Protocols should instruct staff regarding proper handling of sensitive documents in the office, in clinic work areas, and on ambulatory visits, for example. Protocols should also address access of nonauthorized personnel (eg, clients, cleaners) to computer screens and databases.

Electronic access restrictions include password protection, defined levels of access, encryption, and user identification tools (eg, fingerprint scans).

Integrity and Storage

- Original medical records must be unalterable. To correct errors on paper, users should draw a single line through the error; initial the change; and note the date, time, and reason for the change. Software programs should only allow an authorized user to attach explanatory addendums to the existing record. Systems should prevent alterations of original entries. Practices must establish and enforce policies requiring every program user to log in using their own user name to ensure proper identification.
- Create protocols to audit random samples of medical records on a regular basis. This process of reviewing random samples of records provides quality control and is another form of effective risk management.
- Lock up any storage containers or file cabinets that contain medical records. Such storage should be located in areas in the practice that minimize access by nonauthorized persons.
- Back-up EMRs daily, and retain multiple copies of data. Possible data locations include a clinic server, a Web-based backup location, and external hard drives. It is preferable to store backups at off-site and on-site locations.
- Establish and follow a protocol to check the integrity of all backups regularly. Your practice management software program should help you to perform these tasks.

HOW CAN WE CREATE AND MANAGE GOOD MEDICAL RECORDS?

When it comes to medical records, a practice's key resources are its people, IT, and operational processes (**Fig. 4**).

Encourage your practice team to provide input as you are setting up standards, designing protocols, and customizing software related to medical records. As you train your people, remember that knowledgeable staff members make better decisions and that everyone adjusts to change differently. Monitor performance and, when problems occur, re-evaluate and adjust protocols and requirements as needed.

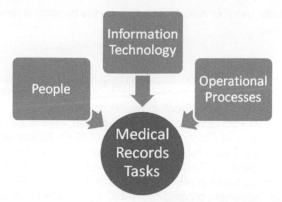

Fig. 4. Key resources for creating medical records. (*Courtesy of* RxWorks, Inc.)

Good practice management software is critical to creating high-quality records. Learn how your software program can help with these tasks, and work with software representatives to customize your program to meet your particular needs.

The protocols or processes you develop, teach to your staff, and use on a daily basis to deal with medical records evolve and change as your practice changes. Protocols should be in writing and available to staff for easy reference. Paper handbooks can work, but guidelines made available electronically are even better for most people.

SUMMARY: WHAT ARE THE LASTING BENEFITS OF QUALITY MEDICAL RECORDS FOR AN EQUINE PRACTICE?

Accurate and comprehensive medical records provide the bedrock of patient, client, and practice information that, along with your professional skills and expertise, allow you to run a successful practice.

It is important to remember that the quality of a medical record is only as good as the quality of the information entered into it, however. As noted by Dr. Gregg A. Scoggins when referencing situations dealing with alleged malpractice, "Veterinary licensing boards, clients, and their counsel, often follow the rule of thumb that if a procedure or task is not recorded in the record, then it was not performed."[6] Thus, we must accept that it is the responsibility of the individual gathering and recording information to enter accurate and complete data into the medical record in a timely manner.

Excellent medical records can enable a practice to:

- Improve the quality of patient care
- Communicate effectively with clients and improve client service
- Educate clients and staff
- Provide key data that can be used to develop better standards of care
- Ease the introduction of new associates and staff
- Reduce liability risk
- Enhance communications with colleagues and increase referrals
- Increase efficiency, productivity and profitability
- Establish procedures and protocols that increase practice value in the event of buy-ins, mergers, and practice sale

Set your standards, use your resources, and reap the benefits of time and effort well spent.

REFERENCES

1. Lacroix C, Clark M. Everyday zoonotics can lead to everyday lawsuits for veterinarians. Suppl Veterinary Forum 2008;25(Suppl A):24. Adapted from Dvork G, Rovid-Spickler A, Roth JA (eds); Handbook of zoonootic diseases of companion animals. Ames, IA, Center for Food Security and Public Health, Iowa State University, 2008.
2. American Association of Equine Practitioners (AAEP). Ethical and Professional Guidelines, Resource Guide and Membership Directory. Lexington (KY); 2009. p. 31.
3. International Association of Electrical and Electronic Engineers, Inc. Definition of interoperability of the National Alliance for Health Information Technology adapted from the Position Statement created for NAHIT by the International Association of Electrical and Electronic Engineers (IEEE), Washington, DC; 2005. Available at: www.nahit.org.
4. Principles of Veterinary Medical Ethics of the AVMA. American Veterinary Medical Association Issues, AVMA Policy. Available at: www.avma.org.
5. Meagher DM. A review of equine malpractice claims. 2005 AAEP Convention Proceedings 2005;51:510–3.
6. Scoggins G. Legal considerations concerning patient medical records. AAEP Convention Proceedings 2005;51:515.

Equine Associate Employment Agreements from the Employer's Perspective

Gerard Lacroix, JD, LLM, DEA Droit Sorbonne, IEP, CAPA[a],
Charlotte Lacroix, DVM, JD[a,b,*]

KEYWORDS

- Employment agreement • Employment contract
- Employee veterinarian • Associate
- Equine veterinary practice • Equine practice
- Employee benefits • Restrictive covenant

An equine associate employment agreement formalizes the relationship between employee and employer. It is a tool. Like all tools, it is suitable for some purposes but not for others. Thus, the first step is to determine our goal, or what we are trying to achieve.

The equine practice owner's objective is to hire and retain qualified equine veterinarian associates who add to the bottom line. Although simple to state, this goal is difficult to attain. Success depends on numerous factors that require different skills to understand, let alone master. Some of these factors, such as "the employment market" and "the economy," are not even under the owner's control.

To realize this complex objective, equine practice owners need to approach human resources globally rather than piecemeal, and certainly not by "winging it." Employers should know how various employee resource tools are utilized and use them in an integrated fashion.

YOUR EMPLOYEE RELATIONS TOOL BOX

Aside from employment agreements, the three other primary tools used to form and implement an employee relations strategy are (1) the employee manual, (2) insurance,

[a] Veterinary Business Advisors, Inc, Countryside Plaza, North, Building E, Suite 1403, 361 Route 31, Flemington, NJ 08822, USA
[b] University of Pennsylvania School of Veterinary Medicine, Philadelphia, PA, USA
* Corresponding author. Veterinary Business Advisors, Inc, Countryside Plaza, North, Building E, Suite 1403, 361 Route 31, Flemington, NJ 08822.
E-mail address: clacroix@veterinarybusinessadvisors.com (C. Lacroix).

Vet Clin Equine 25 (2009) 511–525
doi:10.1016/j.cveq.2009.07.003
0749-0739/09/$ – see front matter © 2009 Published by Elsevier Inc.

and (3) "people skills." Each has its place, and employers need to use all these tools together to retain productive associates.

Employment Agreements

An employment contract is a series of legally binding promises that the employer and employee make to each other.[c] Their primary purpose is to communicate and create accountability. Employment agreements cannot do it all. Employment agreements have two major shortcomings: they are not flexible, and because they are, by their nature, "tools of enforcement," they contribute little toward fostering the cooperative atmosphere necessary for good employee relations.

Employment agreements generally cannot be changed without the consent of both parties. Even if what one party wants to amend is noncontroversial, the other party is inclined to hold that modification as "leverage" for something the other party wants to change. Employees always think that employers can do better (and vice versa). So, when the employer comes, hat in hand, requesting a change to the employment agreement, employees naturally also want to address whatever aspect of their job they want to change.

Negotiating employment agreement amendments can be slow and expensive. Accordingly, items that change frequently, such as an associate's schedule rotation, should not be included in an employment contract. You do not want to have to secure your associate's approval for every change to his or her schedule.

A party who breaches an employment agreement, whether intentionally or not, gives the nonbreaching party the right to seek redress in the courts. Given the costs and burdens of litigation, not all breaches end up in court, of course. A viable claim and the threat of litigation, however, increase the "bargaining power" of the aggrieved party. Ditto a viable counterclaim if the other party threatens to sue you. Because employment agreements are seen as "adversarial" and "confrontational", they cannot form the sole foundation of a positive and cooperative employment relationship (**Box 1**).

Employee Manuals

An employee manual or handbook is a multipurpose document. First, the manual codifies practice policies. Because an employee manual is not a contract, policies can be added, modified, or abolished without employee approval. This gives employers the necessary flexibility to deal with change. Moreover, unlike an employment contract, which is long on commandments but short on explanation, the manual allows employers to explain why the practice rules are what they are. Employee compliance based on an understanding of a rule is usually more effective than fearful obeisance.

The second purpose of employee manuals is to show employees and outsiders that you are serious about your basic responsibilities as an employer. This means keeping a safe and nondiscriminatory working environment that is also drug-, alcohol-, weapons-,[d] and harassment-free. To reduce the risk for incurring liability, including fines and other penalties, practice owners need to show investigators, regulators,

---

[c] Like any other contract in this respect. As an important tool in your human resources tool box, you need to get your associate employment agreement right; however, that is not enough. If you want to retain high-quality associates who contribute to your bottom line, you also need to use veterinarian employment agreements in conjunction with your other employee relations tools. Developing and implementing a comprehensive associate relations strategy is surely burdensome and costly but much less painful and much less expensive than high associate turnover.

[d] Subject to applicable law. Employees cannot be prohibited from bringing their guns to work in some states such as Florida and Georgia.

Box 1
Do you need an employment agreement?

Given the shortcomings of employment agreements, do you even need one?
Not always. In the "good old days," written employment agreements were rare. Employment in the United States is "at will," which means that you can fire your employees at any time for (almost)[e] any reason or for no reason, absent a contrary agreement. Not having an employment contract gives employers the flexibility to modify employment terms as and when needed. Employees can accept the new terms or leave. Even today, many employees do not have employment agreements. Take lawyers, for example. Is it not sweet irony that your lawyer, who is always pestering you to review, revise, or update your equine practice's employment contracts, does not have an employment agreement himself (or for his hired attorneys if he is a firm partner)?

You do need an employment agreement, however, if you want to protect your practice from your employees' actions after they leave. So, more irony, the greatest benefit for employers of employment contracts is realized *after* employment is terminated. Specifically, the contract can prevent your former associate from setting up a competing practice across the street or using all the contacts, know-how, and proprietary information he or she acquired at your practice to solicit (steal) your clients and patients and raid your staff.

Accordingly, the "perfect" employment contract for a self-interested employer would be limited to confidentiality and noncompetition restrictions and prohibitions on soliciting practice clients and raiding practice employees.[f]

Although such arrangements exist, few well-informed and coached equine associates would enter into such a one-sided agreement; nevertheless, there are still plenty who will sign almost anything handed to them and hope for the best.

---

prosecutors, plaintiffs, and courts that they have established policies in all these areas. These policies need to be communicated to employees in the manual. (Of course, none of this does any good unless owners consistently enforce these policies.)

Third, employee manuals are the best place to state the practice's philosophy in a positive way. Employment agreements are not marketing documents. A well-written employee manual presents the practice in a favorable light and helps to promote a good working environment.

Insurance

Equine veterinary employees bring in revenue, but they also increase practice risk. Equine associate risk and reward are often asymmetric. For example, if you send your associate to inject a set of joints in an expensive and well-known jumper, practice revenue increases by hundreds dollars. If the horse dies under your employee's care, potential liability can run to millions of dollars.

Malpractice is not the only significant risk posed by equine veterinary employees. Equine practices are almost all ambulatory, which means that your associates ride about in wheeled weapons each working day. Horses are large and flighty animals, which make them dangerous to themselves and others. Perhaps even more dangerous than horses in some respects, but certainly much more sue-happy, are

---

[e] "Almost," because federal and state antidiscrimination laws prohibit you from terminating an employee because of religion, race, gender, or pregnancy, for example.

[f] Why does not this rationale also apply to lawyer employees? To protect a potential client's freedom to select any lawyer he chooses, attorney professional rules prohibit, and courts do not enforce, a noncompetition restriction when an employee lawyer jumps ship to a competitor (and tries to bring all "his" clients with him). Moreover, attorney-client privilege already prohibits lawyers from revealing confidential information. Law firms would get little benefit from requiring their employee lawyers to sign employment agreements. So, they do not bother.

the clients. They are always bumping into objects and other people; tripping, slipping, and falling; colliding in the facility parking lot; and otherwise causing mayhem. Whenever a practice employee, particularly the "professional veterinarian" is around, clients tend to blame "the expert," who should have "done something" or "known better."

Under the fundamental legal principle of respondeat superior, employers are responsible for their employees' actions that occur within the scope of their employment. When an accident happens, the victim's lawyer searches for an insured party with "deep pockets" to pay for the damage. The insurer, of course, knows this, and therefore peppers his policies with exceptions and other hurdles to avoid paying, leaving the employer with the loss. (If you think that is an overly cynical view of how insurance works, ask anyone with a house in a hurricane state.)

Employment agreements do little to shield the practice from such potential risks. Some contracts provide that an employee indemnifies the employer for his or her acts and omissions, but the employer then has to sue the employee successfully. Employee veterinarians rarely have the resources to pay any substantial damages anyway. To the extent that an associate is involved in any of the foregoing accidents or mishaps, practice owners need to rely on insurance for protection.

People Skills

Perhaps the most influential factor of all on employee morale (and, consequently, employee retention and productivity) is employer leadership (eg, the ability to motivate teams)—in short, people skills.

The following is an example of a related challenge. After being on emergency call "24/7" for 5 years as a solo equine practitioner, you want to hire your first associate. How do you motivate a young associate who puts his "personal" life first yet needs to earn enough to reimburse more than $100,000 in veterinary school debt and support his family?

Materials on leadership and motivating employees fill whole libraries. People skills are so closely intertwined with the subject's personality that they are quasi-innate; thus, it is hard for the relationally challenged to improve. These persons are better off hiring a practice manager with the requisite human relations qualities (**Box 2**).

ANATOMY OF AN EQUINE ASSOCIATE EMPLOYMENT CONTRACT

First, the employer must pay money.

Money

Affording your associate

The basic employer-employee bargain is money for services. Viewed narrowly, this is a zero-sum game. Employers want more work for less money, and employees want the reverse. Each employment party's appetites are tempered by the alternatives offered by the equine veterinary market.

From the equine practice owner's perspective, an associate must not cost more than he or she produces, after factoring in fixed costs and overhead. The best way to approach this is to add up that associate's total cost (compensation plus benefits, including retirement contributions and payroll taxes) and express the same as a percentage of that associate's forecast production.[9] Then compare this number with the maximum percentage the management consultants are saying is tolerable

---

[9] With this number, employers can easily calculate now much additional revenue the practice must generate to be able to afford an additional equine veterinarian.

> **Box 2**
> **Bare naked self-interest**
>
> In this article, the authors repeatedly consider what would be the perfect employment agreement for the employer, what a narrowly self-interested employer would want or do, or, again, the position that an advocate of the employer should take "against" the employees. Equine practice owners must be able to think in these terms when approaching any business situation that requires dealing (ie, negotiating) with people, including their employee veterinarians. You cannot negotiate any matter involving employees without having some conception of what you want; what the employee wants; the extent to which one party's gain is the other's loss; what each of you is (or is not) willing to give up to achieve agreement; and the extent to which a good agreement, a bad agreement, or no agreement affects broader objectives.
>
> You need to establish baselines, or initial positions, with respect to all these points, and imagining what a self-interested employer or employee would want, or how he or she would react to a particular situation, is a good way to start. Using naked self-interest to model negotiations and other business problems is analogous to focusing on the extreme manifestations of a phenomenon to understand it, which is a common methodology in scientific inquiry.
>
> When naked self-interest becomes the only driver of business decisions, however, it becomes self-defeating. As the authors also repeatedly point out in this article, lopsidedly pro-employer employment agreements do not help equine practice owners achieve their objective of hiring or retaining productive associates.

for a "well-managed practice."[h] The current rule of thumb is approximately 25% to 28%, but you actually need to do the information gathering and number crunching for your percentage to be meaningful. Note that it does matter whether you are solely an ambulatory-track veterinarian or an ambulatory practitioner with a referral hospital to support. If the best percentage the equine practice can offer is not competitive with what "well-managed" local equine practices are offering,[i] the practice owner needs to cut costs or increase revenues before being able to afford an additional associate.

To get an idea of large animal employee veterinarian starting salaries, the surveys annually published in *Journal of the American Veterinary Medical Association* are a good place to start.

Commission, base, production

Practice revenue is a variable of course; thus, it is to the employer's advantage to make the employee's cost covary with revenue as much as possible. The less collected revenue the associate generates, the less he or she should be paid, and vice versa. In a simple world, associates would be paid "x%" of their production, period—no base, no benefits, and no expense reimbursement. This scheme is sometimes called "pure commission" compensation, or simply "commission." Although simple, this scheme has adverse tax consequences. There are lost tax deductions for benefits that otherwise would be paid by the employer, and the employer pays payroll tax on salary that would not be paid if the same amount of money was used to pay for an employee benefit, such as insurance.

In the real world, however, a "guaranteed" base salary is fairly typical for equine veterinary practices, particularly for starting associates. In most equine associate

---

[h] Easily found on the Internet. Vetecon.com is a good place to start. "Garbage in, garbage out" is rife in this area, so please pay attention to the assumptions behind the numbers. Hire a good management consultant if you cannot or do not want to do this yourself.
[i] Statistics on this percentage for other equine practices can be found on the Internet.

contracts, the associate is paid the greater of a fixed base salary and a percentage of his production.

Aside from its amount, employers must determine whether the base salary stated in the associate employment contract is truly guaranteed. Many agreements have a mechanism for reducing base salary if an employee's production compensation decreases and stays lower than base for a specified period. Some contracts annually adjust base to 70% to 80% of the prior year's production bonus. Other agreements reduce base to equal production bonus if such a bonus was less than base for the two prior quarters, for example. Most contracts lack this mechanism, however, which means that any substantial lasting revenue decline eventually forces the employer to terminate the associate, because the equine practice can no longer afford him or her.

Production compensation adjusts for inflation, even if imperfectly, but a fixed-base salary does not. That is why some contracts include a base salary escalation clause, which is a fixed percentage[j] or based on the consumer price index. Of course, this escalator clause proves illusory if the contract allows base salary to be lowered to reflect declining production.

Although production-based compensation schemes are not exactly "rocket science," employers still need to ensure that the applicable contract provisions are accurate and coherent.

First, employers need to determine the percentage of gross production to be applied. This may be more than a single percentage. In such "split-rate" schemes, items like specified "low-margin" services or certain product sales earn a lower percentage. In contrast, after-hours emergency and horse show/event duties generally earn a higher percentage. In some plans, the percentages may increase over a sliding revenue scale. For example, the associate receives 25% of all annual revenue he or she generates up to $450,000, 26% for all annual revenue between $450,000 and $650,000, and 28% for all annual revenue in excess of $650,000.

Second, employers must figure out what should be included in, and excluded from, the employee veterinarian's production. Generally, all examinations, diagnostics, treatments, and product and drug sales are included, and all overhead type charges (eg, billing, hospitalization, credit card fees, shipping), in addition to sales tax, and most refills (other than prescription drugs) are excluded.

Finally, employers need to ensure that:

Only services and products personally performed or sold by the employee count for production.

Only revenues actually collected from clients count toward production (thereby motivating associates to help collect the fees).

Base salary is subtracted from the gross production bonus (to implement the "greater of base and production" concept).

All production shortfalls (ie, if production compensation is less than employee's base salary for the relevant period) are combined, and the aggregate deficit is made up before the employee can again become eligible for any production bonus.

Procedures are in place to determine how revenue produced by several veterinarians is shared.

Production calculation, payment, and reporting mechanics actually work.

To preserve flexibility, those items that are likely to change should be consigned to the employee manual.

---

[j] Three percent is currently the most common percentage.

Other compensation

Emergency Equine associate emergency compensation generally means kicking back to the employee all or part of the emergency fee charged to clients, or a higher percentage of the revenue generated by his or her emergency cases.

Horse events A feature unique to equine employment agreements is employee coverage of horse events, such as shows, sales, rodeos, and races. This generates good publicity in addition to producing some revenue; thus, equine veterinarian employment agreements often expressly require associates to cover horse events for additional compensation (usually determined on the same basis as emergency pay).

Miscellaneous Depending on individual circumstances and associate job market pressures, veterinarian employment agreements can include a signing bonus, relocation bonus, board certification bonus (for the new surgeon), and other ad hoc compensation provisions.

Benefits As mentioned previously, it would be easier and less expensive for equine practice owners just to pay associates a commission and require employees to fund their own benefits. These contracts are rare, however, because, first, associates like base salaries and benefits and currently have enough market leverage to force employers to provide them. Second, some benefits, such as health insurance, receive favorable tax treatment if they are offered directly by employer. Third, practice owners cannot get the tax advantages attendant to retirement and certain other benefits unless they are granted to all employees on a nondiscriminatory basis.

Equine practice employers traditionally have offered the same benefit package to every associate on a "take it or leave it" basis. This approach is rather rigid. If an employee veterinarian's spouse is a (human) health worker or a government employee, for example, that associate most likely is covered under his or her spouse's often more generous health insurance policy. The practice's health insurance is of no value to him or her.

A more flexible scheme is to offer an annual benefit allowance of a specified amount (forfeited if not used during the year granted). With this money, associates can buy the benefits they want (subject to the following limitation). A benefit allowance scheme (BAS)[k] should also include a list of required benefits the employee *must* obtain and maintain to ensure that benefits benefiting the practice, such as malpractice insurance, are always in place. BAS employers, however, must "police" the employment contract to ensure that employees have obtained and continue to maintain the required benefits.[l] Thus, if you place your contracts in a drawer and are glad to forget about them, a BAS probably is not for you.

Whether offered as part of a BAS, or in the traditional manner, here are the benefits typically offered at equine practices:

1. Malpractice insurance. Employers have at least as much interest as their associates in ensuring that the associates are covered by adequate malpractice insurance. If, for some reason, the employee's malpractice insurance is unavailable, the aggrieved client is coming after you. Under a BAS scheme, the

---

[k] Sometimes called a flex-plan.
[l] Incredibly, the authors periodically receive calls from veterinarians who have let their malpractice insurance lapse (and are now being sued for malpractice). Employers cannot afford to let that happen.

employment agreement must state that malpractice coverage must be reasonably satisfactory to the employer, or at least specify minimal coverage parameters. Malpractice insurance should include veterinary license defense and be "occurrence based" or include trailing coverage to handle claims that arise after the employee has left. Most practitioners carry malpractice insurance through American Veterinary Medical Association-Professional Liability Insurance Trust (which is currently occurrence based).

2. Health insurance. This is the benefit that employee veterinarians seem to need the most, and many equine practice owners generally offer some form of major medical plan covering their associates.[m] Many contracts include premium caps, however, which means that the associate pays for any premium increase over that amount. BAS employers who believe that proper medical insurance enhances employee productivity ensure that the employment agreement states that health insurance coverage must be reasonably satisfactory to the employer.

3. Retirement. Traditional pension plans (defined-benefit plans) have almost gone the way of the dodo. The burden of saving for retirement has been shifted to employees, who voluntarily fund defined-contribution retirement plans. These plans permit tax-deferred savings with pretax employee contributions. Equine practice owners must grant plan benefits to all practice employees (not just themselves) to qualify for this tax benefit. These programs, which are usually simple individual retirement account and 401(k) plans, can be set up so that employers match all or part of their employees' contributions. To the extent that practice owners want to take advantage of matching, they must also offer it to their employees.

4. Fees and dues. In traditional schemes, equine practice owners generally pay veterinary license fees, Drug Enforcement Agency fees (if needed), and assorted membership dues. These are all required benefits under a BAS.

5. Continuing education allowance. Annual continuing education allowances currently range from approximately $750 to $1500 a year for generalists (up to $3000 for specialists). Equine veterinary employment agreements usually require that an employee's attendance at continuing education events be approved in advance by the employer. With a BAS, any continuing education required by professional rules must be funded with the benefit allowance.

6. Time-off. The usual six major holidays[n] are almost universally paid. As for other leave, equine practices, like their small animal colleagues, show considerable variety. Some practices lump all leave into personal time-off rather than specifying separate maxima for vacation, personal, and sick leave. In the authors' experience, paid leave in equine employment agreements ranges from approximately 5 to 20 days per year (and sometimes increases with employee seniority). Annual paid continuing education leave varies from 3 to 6 paid days. A few practices do not pay for continuing education leave but permit associates to take a specified number of unpaid days. As with an employee's schedule, it is preferable to leave details to the employee manual. Associates must also be informed in the employee manual or elsewhere of leave mechanics: advance notice periods, no carry-forward, the basis on which leave is paid, and the like.

7. Miscellaneous. These are the "trinkets," such as pet supply or care discounts and uniform allowances. Horse supply or care discount trinkets, of course, cost

---

[m] Generally, not his or her family, who usually can be covered under the plan at the employee's expense.

[n] New Years Day, Memorial Day, July 4, Labor Day, Thanksgiving, and Christmas.

considerably more than equivalent items in a small animal practice. Be careful as to how much discount you are giving your employees, because the Internal Revenue Service seems to have taken an interest in auditing such benefits. The general rule is that the discount should not exceed 20% of the regular fee charged to the client.

8. Conspicuously absent is disability insurance. On average, a person is three to five times more likely to be disabled than to die during his or her working years, and equine practice is probably more dangerous than the average job. Despite this, equine practice owners almost never offer disability income insurance, and the authors are not aware of job candidates specifically requesting same (so far).

Equine practice owners must accurately measure and aggregate benefit costs, including retirement contributions, to ensure that they can afford to provide them to their associates. This means that like the practice's insurance policies, the employee benefit plan documents must be studied and understood, regardless of how painful they are to read.[o]

Owners should also determine how specific their employment contract benefit provisions should be. The most favorable benefit provision from the employer's narrow perspective would be limited to the following: "employee will receive whatever benefits package employer offers from time to time."[p] This is not the norm, however, and almost all equine employment agreements continue to list benefits in more or less detail. Because these provisions are legally binding on the employer and cannot be changed without the employee's consent, this is good for equine associates.

Expenses

Unlike small animal associate employment contracts, which rarely address employee expense reimbursement (other than for continuing education), equine employment agreements commonly reimburse employee veterinarians for vehicle and cell phone expenses.

Equine practices generally are ambulatory, which means that associates must use a vehicle adequate for transporting the "box" (ie, the instruments and supplies provided by the practice to treat cases). Equine practices often pass some of the cost of purchasing and maintaining those vehicles on to their veterinary employees by requiring them to maintain a suitable vehicle and, in exchange, agreeing in the employment contract to reimburse such employees at the maximum rates allowed by the Internal Revenue Service (to preserve employer deductibility of the expense).

Equine employment agreements also frequently provide for employer reimbursement of an employee's professional cell phone costs.

Duty

What do practice owners receive in exchange for the money they pay their associates?

---

[o] Employment contracts should provide that plan documents override the contract's provisions, so that the plans can be changed without requiring the employee's approval to amend any corresponding provision in the contract.

[p] Several employment agreements the authors have seen in small animal practice, almost all from the "corporate consolidators," take this approach.

Work

Capable equine associate Although equine employment agreements invariably state that an employee is being hired as an "equine veterinarian", employers don't want just any equine veternarian, they want a qualified, competent, and hard-working equine veterinarian. Accordingly, associates should be fully licensed and not subject to any disciplinary action or investigation for violating any professional rules. They should not be insolvent, so that employers do not have to deal with creditors trying to garnish the employees' wages or be distracted with harassing calls. Finally, if previously employed by another practice nearby, associates should not be subject to any noncompetition or nonsolicitation prohibition that would allow their former employer to sue their new employer.

The employment agreement addresses these matters by having the employee certify that he or she is free of such impediments as of the date of the agreement. The purpose of these "representations and warranties" is less to punish than to force associates to disclose any problems in these areas to the employer before the contract is signed (who can then decide how to address them). To ensure that the employee is aware he or she is making these statements, the employer and employee should read them out loud together.

Duties Listing duties in detail in the employment agreement means that any change requires the employee's consent. Accordingly, the "duty laundry list" (eg, responding to client inquiries within 24 hours) is best left to the equine associate job description in the employee manual. The contract should simply say that the employee will perform all duties reasonably requested by employer in connection with the position of equine veterinarian.

Far more important than the duty laundry list are associate obligations regarding the manner in which associates should perform their duties. Specifically, an employee veterinarian should:

   observe all employer policies that are consistent with his or her employment agreement, whether written or oral, and whether or not set forth in the employee manual;
   perform his or her duties in full compliance with all applicable laws and professional rules;
   contribute his or her best professional skills to the practice (ie, always try hard and never slack off); and
   maintain customary standards of competence and keep up with professional developments

Of the foregoing employee obligations, the first is critical because it links the employment agreement with the equine practice owner's broader employee relations strategy, as implemented by the policies the owner has established.

Schedule The employment agreement must also address the employee's schedule, if only to state average weekly hours and that the employee work in accordance with a schedule reasonably determined by the employer. The contract should also specify the extent to which associates are required to be on-call nights, weekends, and holidays, unless such matters are addressed somewhere else, such as in the employee manual. Other than some basic principles, such as putting the employee on guard that he or she needs to work a flexible schedule, particularly to cover for ill or absent colleagues, or that emergency duties are to be allocated equitably among all (employee) veterinarians, it would be preferable to leave these details to the employee manual.

Exclusivity

In exchange for the salary and benefits, equine practice employers expect exclusivity from full-time associates, such that they do not work elsewhere or otherwise engage in any activity that would interfere with their employment duties (eg, take up too much of their time) or that would harm the practice, including its reputation (eg, organizing People for the Ethical Treatment of Animals demonstrations). Accordingly, associate employment contract exclusivity provisions should be broad in scope.

Confidentiality

All associate employment agreements should have broad confidentiality provisions forbidding not only employee disclosure but any unauthorized use of practice confidential information (which covers many more types of proprietary information than the patient/client information that veterinarians are already required to protect under many state practice acts). The contract should also expressly state that employees must maintain confidentiality and not use any such information for any purpose after their employment terminates. Employers should note that courts routinely refuse to enforce confidentiality provisions unless the practice establishes and enforces procedures (again, in the employee manual) to protect confidential information.

Termination

Employment contract termination provisions are important to end employment relationships that, for whatever reason, no longer fit the goal of "retaining productive associates." Employment agreement termination provisions are divided into two broad categories distinguished by whether or not the terminating party must allege (and, if challenged, prove) a reason for the termination.

Termination without cause

Termination "without cause" or for "no cause" is a misnomer, because no party truly terminates employment for no reason; it is just that the terminating party is not required to provide a reason for ending the contract. Accordingly, an employer invoking this provision can terminate an employee who is no longer sufficiently profitable, or who just "isn't working out," without worrying about having to supply a legitimate reason. Keep in mind that the longer the employee has been hired, the harder it is for a court to believe that the employee was terminated for no cause, and if the employee has a credible "discrimination" story, the employer has the burden of proving otherwise.

Equine veterinary employment agreements almost always adopt one of two no-cause termination approaches. In the first scheme, the contract continues indefinitely, subject to termination at any time by any party with advance notice (usually 30, 60, or 90 days). In the second scheme, the contract renews automatically for a fixed term (almost always one year) unless a party notifies the other before a specified number of days (30, 60, or 90) before the end of the term. The second scheme is far less flexible, because a party needs to wait until the nonrenewal notice period window to terminate the contract. The second scheme can also be dangerous for the employer if, as is often the case, the parties try to renegotiate a new contract after the nonrenewal notice has been delivered. The employee remains on the job during these negotiations, of course, and the old agreement often expires before a new contract is agreed to. If this happens, it is sometimes unclear whether the expired contract's post-termination covenants, such as confidentiality and noncompetition, survive in the event that negotiations subsequently fall through and the associate leaves the practice. The employee argues that the expired contract (including its confidentiality and noncompetition provisions) was superseded by a new oral at-will contract that lasted until he or she left.

In almost all employment agreements, the notice periods or notification deadlines apply equally to both parties; thus, it is not harder (or easier) for one party than the other to terminate the contract. It is unusual, but not unheard of, that the contract provides that the employee must give more advance notice than the employer or that the employee must pay a penalty or forgo compensation if he or she leaves the practice before the notice period has expired.

Termination for cause

Termination for cause allows the terminating party to terminate immediately on the occurrence of certain specified events or for certain specified reasons without bothering with the notice or notice deadline restrictions of a without-cause termination. In virtually all the equine veterinarian employment agreements the authors have seen, only the employer is expressly permitted to terminate the agreement for cause.

"For cause" termination is mostly triggered when the employee does something "bad," such as theft, felony, malpractice, animal abuse, veterinary license revocation or suspension, substance abuse, failure to follow policies, or breach of the employment contract. "Word-smithing" is important here, because the broader the triggers, the easier it is for the employer to terminate the employee. Employers should also consider whether the employment agreement's for-cause termination trigger list is "limitative" or whether an unspecified "good-cause" reason could also allow termination. Not surprisingly, the latter is almost always the case.

Almost all employment agreements also allow the employer to terminate the employee if the employee is disabled and can no longer work for a specified minimum period (after having exhausted all sick and other leave). The minimum period is usually 30 days. Given the rigors and ambulatory nature of equine practice, termination of the equine associate's employment for disability is more frequent than in small animal practices.

After it is over

As mentioned previously, the main advantage for equine practice owners in having an employment agreement in the first place is to subject former employees to post-employment obligations relating to noncompetition and confidentiality.

Noncompetition and related provisions

Noncompetition and related provisions in employment agreements are frequently grouped under the banner of "restrictive covenants." Restrictive covenants include noncompetition and nonsolicitation covenants (in addition to the confidentiality provisions discussed above). A noncompetition covenant prohibits the former employee from competing with the practice within a certain area and for a certain period after his or her employment ends.

Nonsolicitation covenants come in two types, nonsolicitation of practice clients and nonsolicitation of practice employees, which makes talking about nonsolicitation confusing unless you know which type is being discussed. Nonsolicitation of clients means that the ex-equine associate does not contact practice clients to induce them to dump his or her former practice in favor of his or her new employer or the new equine practice he or she has just formed. Nonsolicitation of employees (also called antiraiding or antipirating provisions) means that the former employee does not try to induce employees at his or her prior practice to move over to the competing practice.

States defend free enterprise by almost universally prohibiting contractual provisions that restrain trade, except in certain limited circumstances. In California, this prohibition is absolute and without exception with respect to noncompetition covenants in employment agreements.[q] In most other jurisdictions, restrictive covenants are valid only if they serve to protect what courts generally call the employer's "legitimate business interests" and do not go beyond what is necessary to protect those interests.

In all states, protecting the equine practice's trade secrets and other confidential information is considered a legitimate business interest, and employment agreement confidentiality provisions are almost always upheld so long as (1) the employee could not lawfully have obtained the information elsewhere and (2) the employer actually took steps to protect such information.

Courts have also determined that the "limited to what is strictly necessary to protect legitimate business interests" rationale as applied to noncompetition covenants should translate into the requirement that such covenants be limited in time and space. Accordingly, noncompetition clauses may apply only (1) for a certain period after employment is terminated (most frequently 2–3 years) but not thereafter and (2) in the equine practice's trade area but not beyond. To determine this area, one common method is to draw a circle around the practice facility within which approximately 85% of the practice's clientele is located. Client nonsolicitation covenants should also be so limited in time, but some courts have not required that client nonsolicitation clauses be limited in space, because the relevant activity is "solicitation," which could happen anywhere.

Judicial attitudes to noncompetition and nonsolicitation covenants in employment agreements vary significantly from state to state, with southern and western states generally being more pro-employee than states in the northeast and midwest. Consequently, equine practice owners should obtain comfort from their local contract attorney that the restrictive covenants in their veterinarian employment agreements are enforceable in their home state. The tenor of such comfort depends on whether such state courts agree to modify an offending provision so that it can continue to apply to the former employee in a less restrictive fashion, or if they just void the whole covenant. This so-called "blue pencil rule" is key to assessing the importance of getting your restrictive covenants right the first time. Equine practice owners in states applying the blue pencil doctrine need only ensure that their restrictive covenants are roughly in line with provisions the courts have upheld in the past. If a court later finds that the employer's restrictive covenant was too restrictive, it can ease the restriction(s) to what the court finds reasonable but cannot toss out the whole covenant.

Courts that do not apply the blue pencil rule refuse to fix restrictive covenants they find invalid. According to these courts, employers should be prevented from inserting overbroad restrictions in employment agreements in the hope that employees abide by them, relying on the courts to rewrite the provision so that it remains valid if subsequently challenged. Accordingly, equine practice owners in these states need to pay closer attention to the noncompetition and nonsolicitation covenants in their employment agreements. Specifically, they need to work with their local counsel to:

1. Strictly limit the scope of these covenants to what employers really need to protect their interests. For example, can the employer live with a noncompetition clause

---

[q] Accordingly, employment agreements in California can contain only nonsolicitation and confidentiality covenants.

limited to preventing the former employee from practicing veterinary medicine or being materially involved in the management or administration in a competing practice? Employers should not care if the former employee became a barn hand, file clerk, or groom at the competing equine practice, or simply lent money thereto. Thus, there should be no need for an overbroad clause that would prohibit the former employee from having any association with the competing practice.

2. Be prepared to argue convincingly that the remaining restrictions protect legitimate business interests. At their most extreme, courts in hostile states hold that employers may not prevent their former employers from competing with them. Employers may only prevent ex-employees from using the competitive advantages they acquired at their prior practice to compete unfairly therewith. Trade secrets and confidential information are the most obvious of these competitive advantages, which is why hard-line courts have had little problem upholding confidentiality provisions. To justify restrictive covenants that go beyond what is required to preserve confidential information, employers need to find other convincing competitive advantages to protect (eg, client relationships and practice specific protocols). Note in this regard that hard-line courts are quick to nullify any restriction they judge is not strictly necessary to protect a particular competitive advantage. For example, although even hard-line courts usually accept that former employees should not use the relationships they forged while working at the practice to solicit clients or raid employees, they void employment agreement nonsolicitation covenants that would apply to situations in which such relationships do not exist or are not used. Concretely, this means that such courts (1) only tolerate client nonsolicitation clauses limited to those practice clients the former employee actually serviced during his or her previous employment (because he or she had no relationship with the other clients) and (2) void nonsolicitation clauses that do not permit the former employee to service those practice clients or hire those practice employees who, on their own initiative, have sought out the ex-employee for obtaining veterinary services from, or working for, such an ex-employee.

The foregoing process is arduous and expensive and may not be enough to save your restrictive covenants. All too often, hard-line courts latch on to a superficially plausible reason or precedent for invalidating a covenant they do not like or conclude that clauses are "overbroad" or "unreasonable" without analysis or inquiry.

In addition to the restrictive covenants themselves, equine employment agreements should contain language confirming that the employer may obtain a temporary (and later permanent) injunction preventing the former employee from engaging in prohibited behavior. This is frequently of greater value to the equine practice than receiving a damages award years after the damage is done.

Other postemployment termination provisions

Equine associate agreements could also contain severance payment language, but such provisions are rare. Severance should not be dismissed out of hand, however, because a properly crafted severance scheme could effectively be substituted for a noncompetition or nonsolicitation covenant of dubious enforceability. The former associate would receive a substantial severance bonus, for example, on the second anniversary after employment termination if he or she had complied with contractual noncompetition and nonsolicitation obligations. This scheme should not raise enforceability issues, as with restrictive covenants, but the employer needs to reduce the employee's compensation to "pay" for such severance. Associates may not accept this.

Although not properly a restrictive covenant, including a prohibition in the employment agreement forbidding the parties from disparaging each other is a good idea.

Finally, associates need to be informed of the equine practice's policy regarding postemployment employee references (which should be limited to "Dr Associate worked here from x date to y date"), but this can be left to the employee manual.

Practice Evaluation and Sale Transactions: Preserving Value Through Economic Turmoil

Denise L. Tumblin, CPA

KEYWORDS

- Practice valuation • Practice sale • Profit • Goodwill
- Capitalization rate • Net asset value

The value of a veterinary practice is management's report card and a forewarning of most owners' future financial security.

Dr Hank Autry owns a 4-doctor equine practice in Virginia. Working with his financial advisor, he recently learned that his practice needs to be worth $1,500,000 to be financially secure when he retires in a few years. He knows that he needs to get his "ducks in a row" to be ready for the planned sale to 1 or more of his associates, particularly in the current economy. So he decided to have his practice valued and to learn what he can do to reach his financial goal. (This is a fictional scenario based on real practices.)

Dr Autry is not alone. Even with so much emphasis on the outcome, many practice owners have never had their practice valued. If you had a similar amount invested in your retirement plan, wouldn't you be checking the value everyday? It is time to face the facts; a practice's value is not equal to 1 year's gross, a practice's mere existence is no assurance of value, and the owners' management decisions control the practice's value.

So, let us look at the value of Dr Autry's practice and see how his everyday decisions will control the final outcome.

DETERMINING VALUE

There are several options to value a veterinary practice (market approach, asset approach, and income approach) and several methods within these approaches. Examples of an income-based approach include excess earnings, discounted future returns, and single period capitalization of earnings. A qualified valuator will use his

---

Wutchiett Tumblin and Associates, 3200 Riverside Drive, Columbus, OH 43221-1725, USA
E-mail address: dtumblin@wellmp.com

Vet Clin Equine 25 (2009) 527–535
doi:10.1016/j.cveq.2009.08.003
0749-0739/09/$ – see front matter

or her professional opinion and experience to determine the most appropriate method for a practice situation. This article outlines the excess earnings method for which the principal components of value are net assets and goodwill.

NET ASSETS

Net assets include working capital assets (such as cash, accounts receivable) and drugs, hospital, and retail supplies. Values for these assets are first obtained from the practice's balance sheet prepared on the accrual basis. Each asset is then adjusted from its stated book value to its appraised fair market value. For example, accounts receivable are adjusted to reflect only the value of the collectible accounts. Working capital assets are reduced by working capital debt, such as accounts payable, payroll taxes payable, sales tax payable, and retirement contributions payable.

Net assets also include the practice's tangible assets, such as office supplies, office furniture, medical and office equipment, and practice vehicles. The land and building are included only if the practice owns these assets. Tangible assets are valued at current market value, the price a buyer would pay, given each item's age and condition. Market value can be determined in 1 of 3 ways:

- An independent appraisal by a qualified appraiser who is familiar with veterinary equipment.
- An agreement between the buyer and the seller.
- A financial formula that considers original purchase price, age, and replacement cost.

If real estate is to be valued, obtain an independent appraisal from a qualified appraiser who has experience in valuing special-use facilities. After all assets have been valued, practice debts, such as notes, leases, and mortgages payable, are listed and subtracted from the total to arrive at net asset value.

In primarily ambulatory equine practices (70% plus), the net asset value often represents 50% to 60% of the total value. The percentage is lower in equine referral practices.

GOODWILL

The intangible asset value or goodwill is the value placed on the earnings from operations. To determine goodwill value, earnings generated from the normal ongoing operations of the practice must first be calculated. This calculation begins with practice income as reported on practice tax returns for the last 3 years. Less than 3 years may be included if major changes have occurred, such as the construction of a new facility, the addition of a second practice, severe weather damage, significant growth in revenue (in excess of 20%), and so on.

Practice income is then adjusted to reflect the normal operations of the practice. Adjustments are made for (1) income and expenses that are on the tax return but are excluded from the calculation of value, such as interest expense and the gain on sale of equipment; (2) expenses that are not on the tax return but are included in the calculation of value such as nondeductible entertainment expense; (3) nonrecurring expenses, such as those associated with flood damage, litigation, and relocation; and (4) an increase or decrease in rent expense to reflect the true rental value of the land and building.

An adjustment is also made to the amount paid to owners and associates for their veterinary and management services. This adjustment does not count the number of doctors employed; it considers the medical and management services provided and applies a standard compensation rate to the dollars generated from these services to determine the practice's true veterinary and management expense. In an equine practice, compensation rates depend on how services are provided. Compensation for field-work commonly ranges from 25% to 28%. For outpatient services provided at the practice, the compensation ranges from 20% to 25%, and for surgical services it ranges from 16% to 25%. Management compensation of 2% to 3% may be applied to all revenue generated in the practice. The total plus payroll taxes represents the fair market value of veterinary and management services and replaces amounts actually paid.

The calculated fair market value will be higher than the actual dollars paid if doctors have been underpaid in the short term because of cash flow concerns. The calculated value will be lower than actual dollars paid if owners have been drawing their owner earnings throughout the year in addition to a fair salary for services or if associates have shared in owner profits.

If the practice has developed its own standard for determining veterinary and management pay, consideration will be given to the existing formula.

With income and expense adjustments completed, the expected earnings from operations can be determined for each year included in the valuation. The valuator will then determine the weighted average earnings for 3 years. Many owners worry that the value of their practice is hindered by their strategy of withdrawing all profits at year-end to avoid high corporate tax rates. They are concerned that $0 taxable income means $0 goodwill value. This is not the case.

The goodwill value reflects the practice's ability to generate excess earnings (profit) regardless of whether that profit is left in the corporation or withdrawn. This means that once excess earnings are generated, they can be reinvested into the practice or paid out without reducing the value. Many owners use these earnings to fund their savings; the excess earnings generated not only establish the practice's value but also create investment value outside the practice.

Because the average expected earnings represent the earnings generated by the tangible and intangible assets, the earnings from the tangible assets must be identified and subtracted from the total to arrive at the expected earnings attributed to the intangible assets. The remaining earnings are the practice's excess expected earnings.

Next, the excess expected earnings are capitalized. The capitalization rate reflects the rate of return available in the marketplace from investments expected to produce similar income with comparable risk. There are various methods for determining a capitalization rate. When the summation method is used, the appraiser starts with a low risk rate; US Government notes or bonds are generally considered the benchmark for the risk-free rate. The valuator adds a series of premiums that, in total, reflect the rate of return that an investor would expect to earn by taking the additional risks associated with owning a veterinary practice and finally, the risk associated with owning the named veterinary practice. Historically, the capitalization rate for veterinary practices has ranged from 17% to 33%.

The capitalization rate is then converted to a capitalization multiplier (100% divided by the capitalization rate) and applied to the practice's excess expected earnings to arrive at goodwill value. For example, if a 20% capitalization rate is applied to excess earnings of $100,000, the resulting goodwill value is $500,000:

$$\frac{\$100,000 \times 100\%}{20\%} = \$500,000$$

Looking at it from the buyer's viewpoint, if the buyer requires a 20% return on investment, he or she would want to receive $100,000 in annual earnings from an investment of $500,000.

PRACTICE VALUE

Finally, the values of the net assets and goodwill are added to arrive at the practice's fair market value.

Revenue
- − Normal, ongoing operating expenses
- − Fair market value of veterinary compensation
- − Fair market value of owners' management compensation
- = Expected earnings; calculated as a weighted average
- − Investment return on working capital and tangible assets
- = Excess expected earnings
- × Capitalization multiple
- = Goodwill value
- + Net asset value
- = Total practice value

The buyer and the seller need not obtain separate valuation reports, provided the original report prepared by the seller's valuator fully documents how the value was determined. In this case, the buyer's advisor should review the seller's valuation and comment on differences in opinion or methodology and on how the differences affect the value.

Now, for Dr Autry's practice. The value is currently $850,000.

Net Asset Value	
Accounts receivable	$40,000
Inventory	$40,000
Equipment	$230,000
Total	$310,000
Goodwill value	$540,000
Total practice value	$850,000

INCREASING VALUE

In many practices, goodwill is often the largest component of value. So if the value of your practice falls short of your expectations, increasing goodwill will be the most direct way to increase total value. This means increasing excess expected earnings, which can be accomplished by reducing operating expenses or increasing revenue. Dr Autry's practice value is $650,000 less than his target of $1,500,000. He wants to learn what he can do to build the value and, at the same time, continue to raise his standards of patient care. We began with an analysis of the practice's earnings and capitalization multiple, which revealed that earnings are negatively affected primarily by the practice's fee structure and missed charges.

FEE STRUCTURE

Dr Autry's examination fee is $50, a reasonable level given the economics of his community. His average charge per doctor transaction (ADT) is $170. In well-managed practices, the ADT averages from 4.0 to 4.4 times the examination fee. This means that the doctors' ADT should be at least $200.

We took a closer look at the practice's fee schedule and found that the lameness examination and prepurchase examination fees were low. The practice does have some hospital cases but is not charging for electronic monitoring or hospitalized patient examinations. Several fees for laboratory services, diagnostic imaging, and reproductive services were also low.

We also determined that they were missing charges on a significant number of cases: $40 on 25% of farm calls and $100 on 40% of hospital cases. So, the doctors and staff developed an action plan to reduce the frequency of missed charges.

Making these few adjustments increased the doctors' ADT to $190. This increase will provide more cash flow for doctor salaries, staff salaries, and reinvestment in new technology. Here is the effect on practice value from the increased ADT:

ADT ($)	Practice Value ($)
170	850,000
190	1,200,000

Action step: Is your ADT 4.0 to 4.4 times your examination fee? If not, look closely at your fee schedule. Are your value-based services consistent with other well-managed practices in similar communities? Are you billing for all services provided, including intravenous catheters, assistance at foaling, all injections, and medical progress examinations? Low fees and unbilled services will eventually hinder your ability to provide the best medical care for your patients. As cash flow dwindles, your ability to hire the best and the brightest and to keep up to date with medical technology declines.

OPERATING EXPENSES

I reviewed the practice's operating expenses and found them generally in good order. However, while reviewing the inventory purchases for the previous year, we found an opportunity to change some of their reorder points and to eliminate some redundancy in medications.

Dr Autry reduced his inventory cost from 23% of revenue to 22% for an annual savings of $11,000.

Here is the effect on practice value from the inventory reduction:

Drug and Medical Supplies (%)	Practice Value ($)
23	850,000
22	897,000

Action step: Think lean when it comes to inventory. Target $10,000 to $14,000 of inventory per doctor and a turnover rate of 8 to 10 times per year.

Completing these changes will increase the 1-year value of Dr Autry's practice to more than $1,200,000 within 12 to 18 months. Dr Autry's goal is to maintain his focus to keep his management and medical standards high, his practice operating efficiently, and to continue to improve the value of his practice.

You too have considerable control over your practice's value. If your goals include receiving fair value for your practice and providing the highest standard of medical care, focusing your attention on management and medicine must be part of your plan.

This information is intended to provide the reader with general guidance in practice succession matters. The materials do not constitute, and should not be treated as, appraisal, tax, or legal guidance or technique for use in any particular succession situation. Although every effort has been made to assure the accuracy of these materials,

Wutchiett Tumblin and Associates does not assume any responsibility for any individual's reliance on the information presented. Each reader should independently verify all statements made in the material before applying them to a particular fact situation and should independently determine whether the succession technique is appropriate before recommending that technique to a client or implementing such a technique on behalf of a client or for the reader's own behalf.

Common questions regarding the valuation of a veterinary practice
1. I am hiring a valuator to value my practice. What should I expect in terms of the process?

At Wutchiett Tumblin and Associates, when potential clients call our office, we have a 30-minute conversation to better gauge where they are in their planning process. Questions we may discuss include: What is the purpose for the valuation? When do you want to retire? Who is buying your practice? These answers give us a better idea of how we can help the clients accomplish their goals.

To begin, we send out an engagement letter and document request. The engagement letter states the purpose of the valuation, date of valuation, the assumptions and limiting conditions the engagement is subject to, and the cost to complete the work. The client is required to sign the engagement letter so that the intent of our work is clear to both parties. The document request lists financial information, such as tax returns, financial statements, a depreciation schedule, an equipment list, and an employee census form. We try to make the document gathering process painless.

Typically, we estimate 8 to 12 weeks to complete the report. The client controls the time and cost by the accuracy and timeliness of the information we receive.

When we have received all the documents and information, we start the valuation analysis. Two to three phone calls are scheduled with the client to ask questions and discuss the current operations of the practice. These conversations are critical to the valuator's professional opinion of the practice.

Once we have finalized our analysis and conclusion, we send the client a draft report and schedule a conference to discuss in detail how we arrived at the value. This conference provides an opportunity for the owner to ask questions about the valuation and the next steps involved in the selling process. After the conference, we make the necessary changes and send out a final valuation report.

2. What does a valuation report include?

Introduction and conclusion of value

The introduction and conclusion of value identifies the property to be valued (assets and liabilities or stock), the name and tax structure of the practice entity, the date of the valuation, the standard of value used and a definition of the standard, purpose and intended use of the report, the primary sources of information used by the valuator, assumptions incorporated in the valuation, items that should be brought to the attention of the reader that could affect the opinion of value, the valuator's opinion of the estimate of value, a recommendation to update asset value as of a closing date, and a statement attesting to the independence of the valuator.

Financial information analysis and adjustments

The process for valuing veterinary practices is presented as an overview within this section, beginning with an analysis of the practice's background and history. It describes common scenarios for the veterinary industry and typical ranges for expected earnings. A statistical presentation of certain aspects of a client's practice is compared with published industry information. In addition, it describes balance sheet and income adjustments, as they will be presented later in the report.

Net asset value

This section details the values of all assets and liabilities included in the conclusion of value. Each asset and liability has a footnote explaining the source of the information (eg, tax return, financial statement, representation of management) and all the adjustments made to arrive at the fair market value of those assets.

Goodwill value

The calculation of goodwill begins with practice income and shows every adjustment that the valuator makes in arriving at the earnings stream to be capitalized. Each adjustment has a footnote explaining why and how it was determined. This section also includes the calculation of the fair market cost of veterinary and management services, the return on asset deduction, and application of the capitalization multiple.

Valuation approaches and methods considered and used

Valuation guidelines provided by regulating authorities require a minimum of 3 approaches to be considered when valuing a veterinary practice. This section explains which approaches and methods are considered to arrive at the conclusion of value and then presents the calculated results of each method. A description of the rationale behind the decision to rely on or disregard each approach is provided.

Qualifications and certification

This is a summary of the valuator's qualifications and experience relevant to valuing veterinary practices. This is also the section in which the valuator certifies the conclusion of value, his or her independence, the limiting conditions and uses of the report, and provides the names of individuals involved in the preparation of the valuation report.

Assumptions and limiting conditions

This section details the limiting conditions on the use of the report and on the scope of the valuator's responsibility.

Supplemental information

The remainder of the valuation report contains information considered in valuing the practice. It includes a detailed list of sources of information, historical revenues and expenses, a veterinary industry analysis and outlook, a description of the national economic environment, local and regional demographic and economic environment, and an international glossary of business valuation terms.

3. Does the valuation report need to be updated as of the sale date?

Yes. The fair market value of assets and liabilities should be updated as of the sale date. Goodwill value is constant for 1 year because it is based on a tax year (12 full months of operation).

For example, a practice valuation is completed as of December 31, 2008. The seller and buyer establish a sale date of June 30, 2009. At that time, the assets and liabilities are updated to reflect fair market value as of June 30, 2009. This means completing an actual count of inventory, updating collectible accounts receivable, adding 2009 equipment purchases, and subtracting practice debt. Your valuator should complete the update within a few days.

4. Should I have my practice valued if I am not selling right away?

Yes. A valuation should be viewed as a planning tool. Although the motive is to ensure that when the time comes to sell, you will be fairly paid for the practice you have built, there is a significant fringe benefit. When you go through the valuation process, your attention is focused on the operations of your practice. Because the value of your practice is directly tied to operating efficiency, your attention will result in growing a successful well-managed practice.

5. When are practice valuations mandatory?
   - Buying or selling a practice
   - Buying or selling a partial interest in a practice
   - Writing or updating a buy or sell agreement
   - Planning for financial security
   - Retirement planning
   - Estate planning
   - Third-party financing
   - Mergers
   - Property settlements

6. Why do I need to hire a professional appraiser to value my practice?

   To determine the value of your business, it is important that you hire a professional who specializes in the valuation of veterinary practices. These professionals have extensive experience in the profession and perform their work with objective, unbiased, professional judgment. Valuation is scientific, but it also includes an element of art. It is quite like a surgery. A veterinarian may follow certain procedures as he or she begins a surgery, but the art of surgical skill and experience plays an important role in the outcome. No two surgeries are the same, and the same is true for valuations.

   The valuator is faced with many decisions throughout the valuation process. This is not a task for the inexperienced. An inflated value is of no use when it is rejected by all potential buyers. It can easily result in a seller receiving less than the practice is worth, as overvalued practices that remain unsold for an extended period of time grow stale like overpriced real estate. An undervaluation jeopardizes you and your family's financial security.

   If no valuation is completed and the buyer relies on your representation of value, the liability for misrepresentation falls solely on your shoulders. This can lead to the potential for future litigation.

7. Is taxable income the same thing as excess earnings?

   No. Taxable income is determined for tax purposes as reported on the practice's tax return. Owners of C corporations often express concern about their tax strategy of withdrawing all profits at year-end to eliminate taxes at the corporate level. Because of the adjustment process, they need not be concerned. Adjustments are made to taxable income to arrive at excess earnings, including fair market rent, fair market veterinary compensation for owners and associates, and economic depreciation. Even so, it is best to keep your financial records clean. Pay personal expenses from your personal checking account and business expenses from your business checking account.

8. What makes one practice riskier than another?

   Let us consider staffing, the service or product mix, the facilities and equipment, and transferability as examples. When it comes to staffing, there is higher risk of ownership when staff turnover is high, wages are low, or there are inadequate or nonexistent training protocols. When you consider the service or product mix, there is higher risk associated with a higher percentage of revenue coming from dispensing and retail sales and nonmedical services such as boarding and grooming. Why? Because many of these products and ancillary services can be obtained from sources other than a veterinary practice. With facilities and equipment, owners face higher risk if the building is outdated or is at 100% capacity without the ability to expand because of property constraints. Transferability of goodwill becomes a higher risk in one-doctor, niche practices that are being sold to an outside buyer.

9. Are practice values declining?

The answer is YES if you compare practice value with gross revenue. A historical review of value versus revenue shows startling changes in the age-old relationship:

	Well-managed Practice (%)	National Average (%)
1970s	100	80
1980s	110	70
1990s	80	60
2000 plus	85	50

Caution: The application of a gross revenue multiplier is not a reliable method for determining a practice's value.

The reason for the decline is that owner profit, as a percentage of revenue, is declining. In 1992, the amount available to owners after all operating expenses have been paid and before reinvestment averaged from 18% to 21% of revenue in general equine and companion animal well-managed practices. By 2008, this percentage had declined to 12% to 18%. As goodwill value is tied to profitability, the decline in profit has resulted in a decline in value, as a percent of revenue.

The answer is NO if you look at values in dollars. Dollar values are on the rise in well-managed practices. Owners are paying closer attention to profit variables, such as fees, staff retention, client retention, and advances in patient care. They are also gaining a better understanding of the concept of ownership risk and are putting management systems in place to reduce owner risk for themselves and for future buyers.

To learn more about No-Lo Practice, visit VetPartner's Web site (www.vetpartners. org) and download The No-Lo Practice publication. While you are there, download and complete the No-Lo Practice Threat Advisory Worksheet developed by the Veterinary Valuation Resource Council to estimate your practice's true profitability.

SUMMARY

This article helps readers to

1. Enhance their knowledge about how an equine practice is valued.
2. Learn when a valuation is necessary.
3. Understand the connection between profit and value.
4. Learn the key steps to be taken to improve value.
5. Know what to expect in a valuation report.

Mergers and Acquisitions Involving Equine Veterinary Practices

Brad R. Jackman, DVM, MS[a],*, Owen E. McCafferty, CPA, AVPM, FACFEI[b]

KEYWORDS

- Mergers • Acquisitions • Vision • Corporate structure
- Compliance • Economics of scale

Recently, in corporate America and throughout the world, mergers and acquisitions have been increasingly more commonplace. The pooling of financial, intellectual, facility, and personnel resources in an effort to increase efficiency and reduce expenses has enticed large and small companies. Mergers and acquisitions also allow for immediate expansion and potential diversification. Historically, equine veterinary practices have rarely ventured into this business practice. Companion animal and food animal practices have been more aggressive in pursuing combination of practices. Food animal practices have often combined to accumulate pharmaceutic inventories and avoid duplication of support services, such as billing and collection. Companion animal practices have often grown locally by means of expansion, establishing satellite or separate hospitals; however, more recently, they have also grown through the merger and acquisition processes. For the most part, equine practitioners have viewed themselves as unique and independent, and therefore generally have grown by means of the expansion of services and personnel within their existing practice.

When considering a merger or acquisition, the advantages and disadvantages of combination must be considered. The medical, professional, and economic challenges must all be anticipated, evaluated, and discussed thoroughly. An educated, rather than emotional, decision needs to occur to enhance the possibility of success with a joint business venture.

MERGER VERSUS ACQUISITION

Merger and acquisition are often mentioned together, because the process of combination is often blurred. Acquisition implies the complete purchase of another

[a] Pioneer Equine Hospital, 11536 Cleveland Avenue, Oakdale, CA 95361, USA
[b] Owen E. McCafferty, CPA, Inc, PO Box 819, North Olmstead, OH 44070–0819, USA
* Corresponding author.
E-mail address: bjackmandvm@pioneerequine.com (B.R. Jackman).

Vet Clin Equine 25 (2009) 537–542
doi:10.1016/j.cveq.2009.07.004
0749-0739/09/$ – see front matter © 2009 Published by Elsevier Inc.

organization with the buyer undertaking and imposing all the structural, financial, and management responsibilities on the acquired entity. By definition, a merger is a combination of two companies in which only one company survives and the merged company goes out of existence. Obviously, the difference between the two becomes confusing. Mergers have been further divided into subsidiary mergers, in which the target company now becomes a subsidiary or part of a subsidiary of the parent company, and consolidations, in which two companies merge and form an entirely new company. Thus, the types of mergers are often overlapping and confusing, and that is why merger and acquisition are often mentioned together. In general, a distinct complete purchase of an organization is an acquisition, and any other combination of companies can be considered a merger.

Mergers have also been classified as horizontal, vertical, or conglomerate. A horizontal merger occurs when two competitors combine. This type of merger between large corporations can come under scrutiny related to antitrust grounds if their combination could relate to an increase in market power that could have anticompetitive effects. Most equine veterinary combinations would be a horizontal merger and unlikely to be in violation of antitrust laws, but every precaution should be taken to ensure the legality of the merger. Vertical mergers are combinations of companies that have a buyer-seller relation. An example would be a pharmaceutic manufacturer that would merge with a drug distributing company. These types of mergers are often the most successful, because the companies are involved within the same industry yet have the opportunity to streamline and benefit from the cost savings. A conglomerate merger is the combination of companies that do not have a competitor or buyer-seller relation. Companies consider this type of merger in an attempt to diversify.

STRATEGY FOR MERGER OR ACQUISITION

Companies combine primarily to gain a competitive advantage and to return value to the shareholders. The most commonly stated motives for mergers and acquisitions are to achieve faster growth and to improve the synergies of the company. Historically, equine practice has generally grown through internal growth. This type of growth can be successful but can also be slow and potentially lead to missed opportunity. Combining practices can obviously quickly lead to an increase in growth, but overall growth alone is not a good business practice without enhancing profitability. Synergy to improve efficiency, reduce costs, expand services, and share marketing, for example, should be the ultimate goals to enhance profitability and the probability of the combination being successful.

Distinct advantages in economies of scale can be obtained to improve gross margins and operative profits. Advantages in purchasing of pharmaceutics and supplies, equipment, and insurance, for example, can be obtained. Furthermore, some administrative expenses, such as legal, accounting, marketing, collections, and human resources, can be shared. There also may be the opportunity to share services offered. As the costs related to veterinary medicine continue to increase, any and all cost-saving advantages should be explored and used if feasible. Compliance within the organization is critical to gain the advantage of economies of scale. The business practices of the entities need to be the same, including the computer system integration (practice management and accounting), purchasing guidelines, practice management philosophy, and staff management, to gain the full potential benefits.

Careful investigation, planning, and management are vital for the success of the merged companies. Discussions regarding practice philosophy, goals and vision, ethics, medical practices, organizational structure, leadership, and management strategies have to be the cornerstone of consideration for merger. If agreement does not exist on these basic core values, ideals, and structure, the merger has a high likelihood of failure. In fact, only approximately 20% of all mergers in business are really deemed successful, usually because one or more of these core concerns are not analyzed before the merger.

MERGER IN EQUINE PRACTICE

Equine practice can have multiple potential combinations. Mergers could include two or more ambulatory practices, a hospital with one or more ambulatory practices, a large hospital with smaller satellite facilities, or even possibly one or more larger hospitals. In a simplistic form, ambulatory practices could join to share emergency duty, enhance their purchasing power, share billing and collection fees, and possibly share equipment and technology. These advantages could immediately improve profitability and quality of life. The resistance to the fear of loss of control has to be overcome before achieving the benefit, however. Ambulatory or smaller satellite facilities combined with a larger hospital can have the same benefits, in addition to permitting the ambulatory practice to offer more services to clients, continue to be part of the referral situation, and have hospital specialists serve as an informational resource. The hospital could also be a great source for future ambulatory doctors through its intern program to enhance the growth of the ambulatory practice. These regional relations could generate improved and more consistent medical care, an increase in market share, a cost-savings benefit, an improved quality of life, and an exit strategy for the shareholders. The merger of larger hospitals would not be able to benefit from the more local or regional aspects of the other mergers but could benefit from the enhanced economies of scale, improved operational structure, marketing, and branding and could also provide an exit strategy for the shareholders. Furthermore, all merged entities would gain the aspect of diversification. Spreading the investment over a larger entity would decrease the risk for investment.

DISADVANTAGES AND RISKS WITH MERGERS AND ACQUISITIONS

Most mergers fail because of incomplete research and understanding regarding the companies. Failures are mostly related to inadequate initial investigation, improper planning, or poor implementation. In large corporations, the goal is often to achieve growth to enhance shareholder return quickly. With time, however, the growth and profitability are not sustainable, because the initial research lacked the ability to forecast inadequacies in the design or implementation of the merger. Before entering into a merger, all parties need to be completely committed to the process. It is possible to separate the businesses at a later date if they are properly organized at the onset, but it can be a lengthy and expensive process. A merger should be viewed like a marriage, with the view for a long-term relation.

Chances of success are enhanced if a defined management structure is agreed on and established. This may require a shift in management responsibilities and duties that may be interpreted as a loss of control. For those involved with the responsibilities of implementing the merger process and involved with the management, a great deal of time and direction is required. Shareholders who change their vision or commitment to the combined entity can interfere with implementation of the business structure and impede the progression of the process or the ultimate success of the business combination.

Additionally, in veterinary medicine, client service and perception are vital to success. It is imperative that client service remains a focal point for the practices through the process. The idea of the corporate structure could make clients perceive the new entity as impersonal and only caring about profitability. Good businesses continue to put the client first, which should abate any client concerns.

CONSIDERATIONS AND FRAMEWORK FOR MERGER OR ACQUISITION SUCCESS
Establish Compatibility

As previously mentioned, entering into a merger or acquisition should only be done with due diligence. Goals, values, and medical and business ethics have to be discussed and similar between the companies if the merger or acquisition has any chance of succeeding. Often, a strengths, weaknesses, opportunities, and threats (SWOT) analysis of the businesses is critical to helping making a decision about compatibility and setting a strategy. The strategy should be a plan for fulfilling the unified vision and achieving the strategic objectives. Every shareholder has to be completely invested financially, professionally, and emotionally in the combination.

Leadership and Structure

Any business is only as strong as its design and governance. Strong but unified leadership is a necessity. A defined business plan establishing the corporate structure, management structure, and individual responsibilities should be an initial goal. In larger mergers, a board of directors is formed to guide the business. These members should have good leadership abilities and the vision to propel the business into the future. Officers, such as the president, vice-president, secretary and treasurer, have to be elected or assigned. The officers are actually responsible for the execution of the merger and management of the business. Committees with strong leaders have to be fashioned for the implementation of the merger and management of the business, in addition to serving as drivers for opportunities and development. Time frames for completion and implementation of tasks and systems have to be established and rigidly followed. Compliance and accountability are key components to developing the business structure and enabling the business to achieve its potential.

System Integration

Effective management of a business requires equivalent and consistent data. Combining practices have to agree on the use of a common practice management software and financial management software. The same chart of accounts is necessary, with agreement between the groups on the description and categorization of revenues and expenses. Most veterinary practices are presently on the modified accrual basis of accounting but likely need to convert to a pure accrual-based accounting system. Coding within the practice management software should also be the same to allow for the accumulation of data. This is a difficult process, and it is extremely time-consuming. Additionally, veterinarians are often protective of how they have invoiced, and implementing change often causes resentment and resistance. All parties have to understand that the business is going to have true benchmarking and a far greater chance of success if uniform coding and reporting are instituted.

Outside Consultants or Professionals

Effective and efficient legal and accounting professionals are required to implement a merger or acquisition. Legal and accounting consultants are necessary once the practices involved have been identified; the professional, medical, and personal ethics and goals have been discovered and discussed; and the initial decisions regarding leadership and structure have been made. Accountants help to establish the structure of the combined business and the values of the practices. Attorneys are necessary to draft the documents and to ensure that the laws of the state, commonwealth, or province are followed.

A good attorney and accountant with prior involvement in professional practice mergers are necessary and can be cost-effective. A trained knowledgeable and previously experienced person can anticipate issues that may not be readily apparent. Some governmental entities require specific disclosures before mergers result, including separate filings to attorneys, creditors, and even employees. The structure of the new business, such as a C-corporation, S-corporation, or limited liability corporation, requires input from the accountant and attorney. Disparate compensation plans also need to be addressed with accountant guidance to create a strategy and valuation that is agreeable to all parties involved.

Decisions and guidance are also required on payroll taxes, liabilities, and pension or profit-sharing plans. Additionally, insurance regarding unemployment, worker's compensation, health benefit plans, and liability insurance, for example, need to be addressed. Payroll taxes can be dramatically affected depending on whether the combination is a result of common stock purchase, asset purchase, or merger. Pension or profit-sharing plans may have to be accommodated in addition to other specific plans, such as cafeteria plans, flexible spending arrangements, unreimbursed medical expense plans, and group term insurance. Ideally, uniformity of all plans can be established; however, at the least, they have to be included in the valuation of the entities. Provisions for indemnification of one party or the other in the event of contingent liabilities must also be made. Contingent liabilities include such things as pending lawsuits, losses not known after the transaction date but for which one of the practices was responsible before the valuation date, and income tax assessments after the valuation date as a result of an audit.

The structure of the buy-sell agreement is critical, and there needs to be a provision for buy-out in the event the merger is not successful or a party decides to leave the group. Once practices are merged, they are not easily torn apart. The buy-sell agreement should provide how the party would leave and be compensated in a fair and equitable manner in price, payment period, down payment, and interest rate. Additionally, a noncompete covenant needs to be included that is equal for all parties but does not put any party at risk. Failure to resolve the issue of a buy-sell agreement can be immeasurably difficult if the marriage ends in a divorce at a later time.

LOOKING TOWARD THE FUTURE

As equine veterinary medicine becomes more complicated and expensive, efforts to improve and enhance business practices are paramount. The concept of expanding practices is not new, but the idea of expansion through merger and acquisition is becoming more enticing and commonplace. The basic practices of good business continue to include good customer service, good medical practice, controlling expenses, expanding services, and revenue enhancement. Mergers and acquisitions can be a format for pursing all these goals; the merger structure, governance, and compliance are vital to having a successful venture.

Larger entities have the advantage of economies of scale. Practices with larger gross revenues have greater needs regarding pharmaceutics, medical supplies, equipment, and staffing requirements. Group purchasing, especially with a defined purchasing protocol and agent, can produce better pricing and terms. Increased efficiency of purchasing and inventory can reduce staff and facility expenses, facilitate inventory turns, and reduce wastage. Similar advantages regarding the purchasing and maintenance of medical technology can also be gained. More regional mergers and acquisitions can allow for a sharing of more expensive technology and the related staff and facility costs. At the least, combining orders for equipment can frequently yield a lower purchase price and possibly more attractive financing terms or maintenance contracts.

Better and more accurate business practices can be obtained with combinations by allowing for true and accurate benchmarking. When multiple entities are using the same practice management and financial software, using the same chart of accounts and coding can allow for consistent and timely comparisons. Improvements or deficiencies among the related entities can be rapidly seen and diagnosed by comparison, and steps can be instituted quickly for improvement. Good business practices can then be implemented throughout the entire organization. One no longer has to discover deficiencies and ways to correct them by oneself.

In addition to pharmaceutic and medical supplies, the other major ongoing expense in veterinary practice is staff costs. There are numerous opportunities for potential savings with merged practices. Efficiencies present within one practice can now be shared to be implemented in others. Training programs to effect proficient staff can be shared and possibly occur at different sites. Human resource oversight can be centralized for compliance and company and staff protection. Furthermore, larger staff numbers could allow for better employee benefit plans at a reduced cost. Staff turnover is expensive, and processes that enhance training, provide better benefits, and achieve a proficient and efficient staff attract and retain better employees.

Revenues may be increased by improving the customer experience, effective marketing, adding services and technology, and establishing business practices that allow for proper pricing and collection. A consistent product can be uniquely identified, branded, and marketed. A properly trained and efficient staff can improve the service delivered to the client. Improved technology and additional services enable more thorough medical care, which can enhance revenue and improve client service. Superior business practices can minimize missed charges and develop more effective collection policies. Additionally, combining practices may solidify or garner more market share, which should translate into increased revenues.

SUMMARY

Combining practices can be professionally and economically advantageous but requires a great deal of thought, planning, and implementation. Do not be surprised if things that have not been anticipated suddenly appear. When two individuals or entities join together, the variances and difficulties can be extraordinarily unique and creative. Try to anticipate as much as possible, as soon as possible, to enhance the possibility of success and avoid hard feelings. If due diligence is performed and true business teamwork is undertaken, the benefits can be enormous and rewarding.

Erratum

An error occured in the article "Prognosticating Equine Colic," by Sarah Dukti and Nathaniel White, Volume 25, Issue 2 (Augest 2009), on pages 223 and 224 regarding survival rates. In **Table 2** on page 223, under Freeman, 2005,[68] the short-term survival rate for Strang SI is 89%, not 64%. The corrected table is reprinted below.

This error is also on page 224, in the 12th line of the first full paragraph. The correct sentence should read, "In 2005, Freeman and Schaeffer[68] reported on 157 horses with strangulating lesions of the small intestine and reported short-term survival to be 89%."

Vet Clin Equine 25 (2009) 543–544
doi:10.1016/j.cveq.2009.08.004
0749-0739/09/$ – see front matter © 2009 Elsevier Inc. All rights reserved.

vetequine.theclinics.com

Table 2
Survival statistics for diseases

Small Intestine	Type	Survival (%)
Freeman, 2000[25]	Simple versus strang	Simple (91) Strang (84) Long-term (68)
Fugaro, 2001[64]	R&A SI	Short-term (65) Long-term (47)
Van der Boom, 2001[65]	Staple anastomosis	Short-term (50) Long-term (61)
Semevolos, 2002[66]	SI	Short-term (88) Long-term (57)
Freeman, 2005[68]	Strang SI	Short-term (89)
Mair, 2005[22]	SI	Short-term (75.2)
Stephen, 2004[67]	SI Volvulus	Short-term (80)
Archer, 2004[69]	Epiploic foramen	Short-term (69)
Garcia-Seco, 2005[26]	Lipoma	Short-term (60) Long-term (64)
Freeman, 2005[68]	Epiploic foramen	Short-term (95)

Cecum	Type	Survival
Plummer, 2007[75]	Cecal impaction	Medical Tx short-term (81) Surgical Tx short-term (95)
Martin, 1999[76]	Cecal intussusception	(83)

Large Colon	Type	Survival
Ducharme, 1983[77]	LI LI impaction LI impaction	(56.7) Surgery (58) Medical (95)
Phillips, 1993[28]	LI	(80)
Mair, 2005[22]	LI	(89)
Hassel, 1999[79]	Enterolith	Short-term (96.2) Long-term (92.5)
Granot, 2008[81]	Sand	Short-term (100)
Hardy, 2000[82]	Nephrosplenic	Short-term (92.5)
Huskamp, 1983[83]	RDD	Short-term (100)
Harrison, 1988[84]	LCV	Short-term (34.7)
Snyder, 1989[85]	LCV	Short-term (36) Short-term 270 deg (71)
Southwood, 2002[86]	LCV	Short-term (68) (1998–1999)
Embertson[87]	LCV	Short-term (83)

Small Colon	Type	Survival
Ruggles, 1991[102]	SC impaction	Long-term medical (100) Long-term surgical (39)
Frederico, 2006[104]	SC impaction	Short-term medical (91) Short-term surgical (95)
Dart, 1992[35]	SC R&A	Short-term (100) (4 horses)

Abbreviations: LCV, large colon volvulus; LI, large intestine; R&A, resection and anastomosis; RDD, right dorsal displacement; SC, small colon; SI, small intestine; strang, strangulating; Tx, treatment.

Index

Note: Page numbers of article titles are in **boldface** type.

A

Acquisition(s)
    equine practices and, **537–542**
        considerations and framework for, 540–541
        disadvantages of, 539–540
        future related to, 541–542
        risks associated with, 539–540
        strategy for, 538–539
    merger vs., 537–538
Action plan, in CRM, 472
Ambulatory practice, design of, **489–498**
Assets, net, of equine practice, 528

C

Compensation, in equine associate employment agreement, 514–519
Confidentiality
    in equine associate employment agreement, 521
    of medical records, 506
Core values, establishment of, 459–460
Cost(s), CRM–related, 472
CRM. See *Customer relationship management (CRM).*
Culture, of organization, 486–487
Customer buying behavior, understanding of, in CRM, 472
Customer relationship management (CRM), 467–473
    action plan in, 472
    area demographics in, 471
    costs of, 472
    described, 467–469
    internal "self-evaluation" in, 471
    monitoring in, 472
    practice goals in, 469–470
    professional goals in, 469–470
    strategic plan in, 472
    tactics and tools in, 472
    target market in, 471–472
    understanding customer buying behavior in, 472
Customer service, in equine practice, **421–432**
    client experience, 425–429
        described, 425–426

Moving?

Make sure your subscription moves with you!

To notify us of your new address, find your **Clinics Account Number** (located on your mailing label above your name), and contact customer service at:

Email: journalscustomerservice-usa@elsevier.com

800-654-2452 (subscribers in the U.S. & Canada)
314-447-8871 (subscribers outside of the U.S. & Canada)

Fax number: 314-447-8029

Elsevier Health Sciences Division
Subscription Customer Service
3251 Riverport Lane
Maryland Heights, MO 63043

*To ensure uninterrupted delivery of your subscription,
please notify us at least 4 weeks in advance of move.

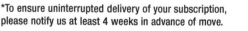

Printed and bound by CPI Group (UK) Ltd, Croydon, CR0 4YY

03/10/2024

01040463-0011